From War to Work

Drug treatment, social inclusion and enterprise

Rowena Young

The Foreign Policy Centre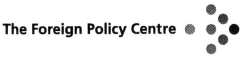

Globalegacy

First published in 2002 by
The Foreign Policy Centre
The Mezzanine
Elizabeth House
39 York Road
London
SE1 7NQ

Email info@fpc.org.uk
www.fpc.org.uk

ISBN 1-903558 07 7

Cover by David Carroll

Typesetting by John and Michael Breeze

The Foreign Policy Centre

www.fpc.org.uk

The Foreign Policy Centre is an independent think-tank committed to developing innovative thinking and effective solutions for our increasingly interdependent world. We aim to broaden perceptions of what foreign policy is, revitalise public debate about foreign policy goals and find new ways to get people involved. The Foreign Policy Centre publishes books and reports, organises high-profile conferences, public lectures and seminars, and runs major in-house research programmes on cross-cutting international issues.

For details of current and forthcoming publications, please see the back of this pamphlet. Individual publications should be ordered from:

Central Books, 99 Wallis Road, London E9 5LN
T +44 (0)20 8986 5488 F +44 (0)20 8533 5821

To order online go to www.fpc.org.uk/reports. For further information about the Centre, including subscriptions, please visit our website or contact us at info@fpc.org.uk

Globalegacy

Globalegacy is a UK-based humanitarian corporation dedicated to the economic and social development of impoverished urban communities within the G-20 countries. It is mobilizing alliances of corporations, governments, NGOs, foundations and universities to invest their money, people and ideas collectively and over a ten-year period into these communities. These investments will be catalysed through a portfolio of commercial and enabling ventures (Investment Fund), on-the-ground experts (Externship Programme) and local resources (Do-tank). For more information please visit www.globalegacy.cim

About the author

Rowena Young is Development Director at Kaleidoscope, the UK's leading one-stop drug treatment agency.

She established **simplyworks** in 2000 – a government-supported pilot social enterprise creating jobs for unemployed as well as long-term drug users. **simplyworks** is currently being spread across the UK. Previously Rowena worked in journalism and at the think-tank Demos. She is a trustee of Children's Express and is on Centrepoint's advisory board. She is a member of the Community Action Network and Vitamin-e.

Rowena can be contacted at r.young@can-online.org.uk.

Further information about **simplyworks** can be found at www.simplyworks.co.uk

From War to Work

Drug treatment, social inclusion and enterprise

Preface and acknowledgements

Though ideas are most often credited to individuals they usually result from the generous deliberation and investment of numerous others. Support for the development of the ideas in this report has been unstinting.

Several people have been key: Martin Blakebrough at Kaleidoscope has been a worthy advocate of holistic approaches to drugs and first encouraged me to look at the Asian examples; Luke Samson, Forum's chair, enabled me to travel to Asia and see the work of Forum members; Luke and Martin, together with Tariq Zafar, Shobha Kapoor and Neville Selhore and many staff and participants of their projects have critically explained and discussed their work at considerable length, have been inspiring in their commitment and boundless in their hospitality; in commissioning this report, Mark Leonard and Sunder Katwala at The Foreign Policy Centre have been exemplary in helping to build the bridges between practitioners, their clients and policy makers, and facilitate the exchange of ideas between parts of the world that rarely learn from one another; Craig Cohon of Globalegacy has been a model sponsor – exact in his analysis, quick with his support and a keen enthusiast for taking the agenda forward.

I am grateful to Mike Trace, Richard Wilkinson and Polly Toynbee for spirited debate of the report's main arguments at an early seminar and to them and Eric Blakebrough, Rosalie Chamberlin, Moira Wallace, Ben Jupp, Sophie Linden and officials at the World Health Organisation for perceptive comment on a draft. Of course, the views the final report contains remain my own.

Three further individuals have been a great credit to The Foreign Policy Centre – Phoebe Griffith for ably taking the overall organisation in hand, Rachel Briggs for pointing up unexplored angles and Rob

Blackhurst for taking the report to all the relevant audiences. Thanks are also due to the Centre's team of interns, particularly Conrad Smewing and Maria Moorwood.

I have benefited from many hours' work at the Community Action Network's Mezzanine and am thankful to its director Adele Blakebrough who was bold enough to suggest the idea of a report to The Foreign Policy Centre in the first instance.

Finally, and not least, I owe much to the staff and clients at Kaleidoscope and **simplyworks**. Their stories and reflections provided the original impetus to look beyond the usual responses to drugs and I hope this report plays some part in making their job easier.

Rowena Young

London, March 2002

Foreword by Globalegacy

The damage is done. The symptoms and causes are known. The solutions exist. But no one has yet articulated a coherent vision that effectively addresses problem drug use. It is time for a new approach to helping those whose lives are destroyed by drugs.

From War to Work: drug treatment, social inclusion and enterprise demonstrates that the current approaches to drugs policy are having little if any long-term effect; in fact they may even be making the problem worse. It proposes a strategy for reform that would focus on those most at risk and treat them as more than criminals or patients.

The report clearly and rightly asserts that the war on drugs has failed because we have segmented the drugs problem into legal and medical components, and then offered one-off solutions to each. No one has addressed the links between the social, economic and cultural factors that trap drug users in cycles of crime, poverty and illness. Taking examples from grass-roots projects in Asia **From War to Work** proposes a more holistic approach to treatment, training and employment.

Drugs are an old problem and the debate surrounding them is complicated by out-of-date fears and prejudices. Creating new and innovative systems to effect profound change in the drug debate is a pressing necessity. Unfortunately, a lack of collective leadership and shared vision prevents politicians and experts from exchanging their knowledge, learning from each other's work and implementing new solutions. It is time for collective leadership, for legislative, political and social enterprise organisations to come together and serve one shared purpose.

This coherent and comprehensive report offers hope for the future of our local and global communities, and a vision of how drug use can be safely and sustainability managed. Let us hear the call.

The Globalegacy Team

London, March 2002

1. Executive summary

Problem drug use is getting worse. After decades of crackdowns most indicators point to rising levels of drug use, even more rapidly rising levels of drug misuse, and a worsening death rate.

Problem drug use is not a mystery. There is now a large body of evidence on its causes. Although drugs are used by people from all backgrounds there are strikingly close correlations between the most problematic forms of drug use and social exclusion. Growing inequality and deprivation in the 1980s and 1990s has fuelled a dramatic worsening of the drug problem.

Partly because they failed to tackle these causes law enforcement remedies have consistently proven ineffective at best, counterproductive at worst. However, alternative methods have not turned out to be panaceas either. The growth of medical treatment to tackle addiction has a better track record than law enforcement, but has been only partially successful because of a limited view of why people misuse drugs.

People's propensity to use drugs in problematic ways is best understood in terms of five key causes: access and availability; alienation; loss; a lack of alternatives; no future prospects. Together these factors go a long way to explain both who becomes a dependent drug user, and why the numbers have risen so sharply in recent years. The environmental causes of these five factors are all currently favourable in the UK: increasing availability because of the combination of abundant supply and effective distribution networks; alienation as the traditional bonds of family, community and work weaken; unstable and often abusive families; social exclusion and long-term unemployment in some communities.

It should be obvious that successful policies need to address all of these causes. Yet debate, and practice, in most of the Western world has been distorted and held back by an often hysterical climate that has made it hard to face the facts head on.

Fortunately, while debate in the West has been frozen or polarised between prohibitionists and advocates of legalisation, projects elsewhere in the world have turned their attention to the practical measures that can reduce problem drug use. At the forefront of this work are a group of projects in Asia that have responded to the world's worst drug problems by developing more holistic methods of dealing with these causes. Many of these are brought together in the Forum network. Their work combines treatment and counselling with a much more concerted emphasis on skills and creating jobs for their clients. All are highly pragmatic – concerned above all with the outcomes they achieve rather than being attached to particular methods or professional traditions.

That we should be learning from drug projects in Asia underscores how much has changed while policy has stood still – drug use as well as production is now a truly global phenomenon. Their work points to the need for drug policy in the West to take a radical turn if it is to be more successful in the coming decades than it has been in the recent past. These are some of the key recommendations:

- There needs to be a change in the tone of the debate – to focus on outcomes not fears and prejudice.

- The key to better outcomes is to address causes – not symptoms. These causes include social as well as personal factors.

- We need an holistic approach – in which work is key. Treatment has a role – but all the key causes of addiction need to be tackled, not just medical ones, if people's lives are to be changed.

- Since social enterprise offers one of the most effective ways of promoting lasting change in people's lives – and reducing the numbers at risk of developing problem use – it should play a central role.

- Sorting out the law on drugs is a necessary but far from sufficient condition for reducing the harm caused by drugs, although there are practical steps which could be taken now to prepare the way for a new legal framework.

- New domestic policies need to be matched by a more active global approach to tackling the causes as well as the symptoms of the drug problem.

- We need to ensure lessons are learnt – this is one field where a lack of talk costs lives.

This pamphlet makes the case for moving the current debate forward. At the moment one side focuses solely on drugs supply – believing that if only it could be stemmed the problem would be solved. The other focuses solely on the drugs themselves – believing that if only their legal status could be changed the problem would disappear. This pamphlet shows why both are wrong, why people, not drugs, lie at the heart of the drug problem, and why the only lasting solutions will be ones that address the personal and social factors that make people dependent.

2. Introduction: Why we need a new approach to drugs

Drug policy in the Western world stands out as a story of continuing, almost unmitigated failure. While other problems, from unemployment to youth crime, have proved amenable to serious debate and imaginative solutions, drug policy sometimes appears frozen – a victim of an unhealthy cocktail of acute public anxiety, simple nostrums, tabloid bile, vested interests and political opportunism.

The damage done

Since drug consumption in the UK first came onto the legislative and public policy agenda at the beginning of the twentieth century, the number of people affected by drugs has steadily increased. And while drug use remains only one of many causes of self-harm – alcohol causes around ten times and smoking around thirty times more premature deaths every year than drugs – the detrimental effects of drugs tend to be more acute and are becoming rapidly worse.

The fact that a majority of under 25s are now recreational drug users is not in itself a problem. The vast majority are able to use drugs, even the so-called hard drugs, without long-term damage. Most simply grow out of them. Our concern here is that since the 1980s, problem use has grown faster than ever before, though it is almost certainly consistently under-reported.

What should most worry policymakers is the collateral damage caused by the sheer scale of the drugs industry and by the impact of drugs on the many who cannot cope:

- the rising number of problem drug users;

- the lengthening life cycle of self-harm;

- the declining age of first use;

- the rise in drug-related deaths and ill-health;

- the pernicious nexus of social exclusion and drug misuse, particularly where it is most concentrated in some communities;

- the role of criminal convictions for non-violent drug offences in undermining efforts to rehabilitate drug users;

- the extent to which the drug economy fuels acquisitive and organised crime domestically, as well as internationally;

- and the close links between the drug trade and oppression, which has become starkly apparent once again, now that the war in Afghanistan has highlighted the country's central role in the world heroin trade.

A polarised debate

In the past the abundant evidence of the harms caused by drugs has sometimes done more to close off debate than open it up. Yet drug policy could be about to become interesting. The Anglo-American tradition of drug policy that has shaped the response of industrialised nations for many years now stands at an impasse. On one side stand the advocates of a continuing war on drugs. For them psychoactive substances are intrinsically evil. Almost no price – in money or civil liberties – is too high to pay to stop the traffic of drugs or their sale by immoral dealers to misguided consumers. On the other side stand the increasingly vocal advocates of treating drug addiction as a disease, a problem of health rather than law enforcement, who pour scorn on the prospects of curbing the availability of drugs and point out that no society in human history has abjured all use of psychotropic substances. Their argument is that, as with alcohol, the best we can do is to provide help to those individuals who cannot control their own use.

At the moment the tide is with the second group. But neither can claim to have had much success in preventing a steady upward trajectory in the scale of problem drug use. The most recent figures show, if anything, that the situation is becoming more acute. In 1998, there were nearly 3,500 drug-related deaths in Britain, a rise of 19 per cent in four years. The number of problem drug users is doubling every four years: there are currently around 270,000 registered drug dependents – 540 times the number registered in the Sixties. For some the cycle of dependency is becoming lifelong, and treatment agencies face the prospect of developing services for the elderly. The age of first use is falling and the largest ever cohort of 20 to 24 year-olds (58 per cent) now report having used illicit substances at some point in their lives.

Judged by any objective criteria, the prohibitionists have a particularly bleak track record: in the US and UK there is not a single piece of evidence to show their interventions work. Given enough investment of resources seizures can grow impressively, but the quantities of illicit drugs hitting the streets show an unerring ability to keep pace – at an estimated ratio of about ten kilos reaching the streets for each one that is seized. Today, levels of heroin entering Britain make it the only western nation to feature in the world's top five heroin importers; the drug is becoming purer and there is evidence it is newly available in communities which in the past had been free of supply. £10bn of acquisitive crime is carried out every year in pursuit of the money to pay for it all. Research by the University of York estimates the economic costs of drugs at between £6.7bn and £6.8bn (combining health, criminal justice and benefit costs).

Oscillations in drug use and related crime have more to do with demographic factors, shifting fashions for particular drugs and generational cycles of attraction and revulsion, than they do with policing. The one certainty is that drug policy itself has had little, if any, positive effect. Moreover, although governments are beginning to be more selective, to date the patterns of police behaviour and arrests have given purveyors of hard drugs the easiest ride. In recent years, more than 90 per cent of drug offences in the UK, for example, have been for possession, and three quarters of those involved cannabis (although this is finally set to improve now cannabis is being reclassified). Both here and in the US the war on drugs has been a resounding failure. Rarely in the history of wars have so many achieved so little at such a high cost.

The treatment world does at least have sound foundations. The National Treatment Outcomes Research Study (NTORS) which was conducted through the Nineties and is the largest ever of its kind in the UK, concluded that 'treatment works', though its authors were quick to stress that this headline comes with many caveats and is no grounds for complacency. By its nature, treatment – advice, counselling, prescribing and alternative therapies – succeeds in attracting those whose drug use poses the greatest health and social problem. Recreational users by contrast rarely perceive themselves to have a problem.

Treatment can reduce harmful behaviour, improve physical and emotional health, and help cut drug-related crime. But its ability to transform the features of a person's life that led to dependent drug use is doubtful – it's not uncommon to find clients who have been round the treatment loop a dozen times, and conservative accounts suggest around two thirds of treatment excludes or fails – if you count abstinence from uncontrolled use as your goal. Some studies suggest relapse rates are in fact as high as ninety per cent. Just as important for the future, the treatment providers have made no in-roads on the groups at risk of debilitating use. Every year more join their ranks. An honest end of term report card might read: 'could do better'.

A new radicalism in Europe and Australia

Across Europe, governments have acknowledged past failures and are now developing interesting new approaches which are taking them further away from the American tradition. The Swiss are taking the idea of addiction-as-illness to its logical conclusion and experimenting with large scale heroin prescribing for users to inject under supervision. Unthinkable in the UK in the current climate, public referenda in the cantons to be affected by the trials, returned a two-thirds majority in favour of the initiative. Meanwhile, the Portuguese government is bringing addicts in from the cold with a far-reaching decriminalisation of drugs, including heroin.

The Government of Western Australia under Premier Geoff Gallop has created the environment for greater pragmatism in social policy by holding public hearings on contentious subjects including drugs. Last year experts prepared background papers drawing together evidence on all the issues, then met with a cross-section of the general public, policy makers and politicians to review current policy. Over a week of intensive debate, delegates voted on recommendations. All the workings were posted on the web. Though not formal referenda, these exercises indicated strong support for new lines of action. In Perth, the public unequivocally backed the introduction of proper treatment for teenagers, highlighted necessary links with wider economic and social policy and pushed for greater emphasis on vocational training and work.

In the UK such radical moves remain largely off the agenda. Instead we have settled for a more conservative 'balanced approach', which essentially involves matching higher spending on law enforcement with higher spending on treatment. Scotland has started to show where devolution may lead to interesting policy departures: already the new government has added employment for drug users as a fifth column in its national strategy and set up an Effective Interventions Unit to research best practice and develop policy. South of the border, some senior members of the Cabinet are still more inclined to play to people's fears when they talk about drugs than to appeal to the facts. In issuing more positive guidance on heroin prescribing and recommending re-classifying cannabis, the Home Secretary has sent a powerful signal that the government is newly prepared to listen. But introduced unilaterally, even the success of evidence-based reforms like these, and the political fortunes of their sponsors, remain vulnerable to the vagaries of public prejudice and condemnation.

In the long run it may turn out to be unwise to act without a full public debate. The forces opposed to change remain strong, and have in the past been able to sidestep the need for evidence and soundly based argument.

Drug misuse as a social as well as an individual phenomenon

The advent of new approaches to policy are to be welcomed. But in the main they still represent little more than tinkering, founded on a fundamentally limited conception of the problem. At root, problematic drug use and serious supply are still treated by clinicians and criminologists respectively as symptoms of personal pathology. This is despite the fact that since the 1980s, the profile of dependent drug users in the UK has taken a profound shift and now correlates overwhelmingly with the socially excluded on the sharp end of growing socio-economic inequalities. Many of the consumers in what is now the world's third largest industry do not suffer much damage to their lives, or chronic addiction. But for those whose lives are damaged, all serious analyses of the epidemiology of their use suggest that a wider public health approach which encompasses the full range of tools of social policy is more likely to work than either punitive legislation and isolated arrests on the one hand, or treatment alone on the other. An emphasis on more constructive livelihoods would be likely to redirect producers' efforts too, changing the dynamics of drug markets for good.

The good news is that there are clues to a happier way forward. They can be found by looking not to the West but to the East. In Asia a new generation of more holistic, enterprising models of drug treatment, brought together in the Forum network, are attempting to address the structural issues, as well as the personal ones, that lie behind their clients' difficulties. Their central insight is that sustainable progress depends on dealing with all of the different factors – ranging from the physiological to the social – that can cause addiction. Specifically, that means helping drug users to find new networks of support, providing them with skills and jobs, and revitalising the communities they come from, as well as helping them to fight physical and emotional dependence.

Where this is done effectively there is a double dividend: on the one hand a reduction in the risk of relapse, and on the other a stemming of the flow of new users. For projects working in areas of cultivation there is a third dividend, as poor farmers find alternative sources of income and thus curb the supply to the cities and international drug rings.

Perhaps the most distinctive feature of these new organisations (such as Nai Zindagi in Pakistan, Mukti Sadan in India, or Pink Triangle in Malaysia) is that they see themselves as economic enterprises, as well as social or health ones. By creating jobs for their clients they have also found a way to generate income for themselves through everything from reconditioning jeeps and building environmentally-friendly houses, to selling condoms to sex workers and running light industry. As a result they are highly cost effective, particularly when the long run costs and benefits are taken into account.

The globalisation of drugs

That we should be looking to Asia for lessons on drugs underscores how much has changed. As little as ten years ago the world could still sensibly be divided into countries that produced drugs and other countries that consumed them. Debate revolved around whether to cut supply at its source or to reduce demand in the West. More recently it has become clear that this divide is anachronistic. The main producer and distributor countries also face chronic problems of drug misuse among their own populations. At the same time production in the West – from Switzerland to Oregon – has sharply increased, whether of cannabis or pharmaceutical drugs. In the US, home grown meta-amphetamines, a more potent kind of speed, are the fastest growing drugs in circulation and in the UK, Department for Trade and Industry analysts predict that it will steadily become easier to manufacture a wide range of synthetic drugs using portable technology.

The relevance of Asia stems from this new reality. Pakistan and India have developed new answers to the challenges we face because they are now home to some of the world's largest populations of problem drug users – over 1.5 million in the case of Pakistan – as well as being producers.

Sadly, the prosperous developed world has in the past rarely been good at learning lessons from the South – despite isolated exceptions like the Grameen Bank which has now been copied in cities all over the Western world. However much the US model fails, and however many billions continue to be squandered, there is always a long queue of experts, pundits and commentators eager to advocate its virtues. When it comes to drugs, even the most highly educated sometimes appear happy to leave their critical faculties behind and cling to the child's view of the world as a simple battle between the good guys and the bad guys.

Propitious times for a new approach

Why then should we be optimistic? There are four main reasons why the timing may be propitious for a major step forward in how we think about drugs in the UK.

The first is that the tone of debate is now changing – partly because the financial and social costs have become intolerable, and partly because the public has lost faith in strategies that often seem to be at odds with the evidence and their own experience and priorities. As the European and Australian experiments gather speed, it is hard to see how the genie can be put back in the bottle.

The second is that practice is taking the first steps to catch up with the evidence. The UK government and the Scottish Executive have just launched employment programmes for drug dependents and are beginning to see the links between treatment and regeneration. Other European governments are trying to deal with drugs in a humane and pragmatic way. Organisations like the Merchant's Quay Project in Dublin and Kaleidoscope in London integrate treatment with education, jobs and resettlement, and the more thoughtful policy experts are starting to acknowledge that this is one field where holistic approaches are a necessity rather than a luxury.

The third is that policy-makers are beginning to understand that there is no longer any boundary between domestic and international policy where drugs are concerned. Success in tackling other global issues, from climate change and terrorism to inequalities between the North and South and migration, through broad international alliances, provides grounds for confidence that some of the same tools could be applied to drugs.

The fourth is that a new alignment of institutions is taking shape that could prove much more effective than what has gone before. The new National Treatment Agency, responsible for fostering more and better services for drug users, will be critical. Just as important will be the Employment Service which is now for the first time thinking about helping long-term drug users, the Neighbourhood Renewal Unit and Local Strategic Partnerships which are dealing with drugs as part of their wider efforts to regenerate communities, the police who are in some cases leading the argument for a sharper focus on dealers of hard drugs and more enabling approaches for users, and the Youth Justice Board which has proven the effectiveness of targeted approaches for young people at greatest risk of perpetuating their exclusion through worsening cycles of crime.

The drug debate is finally starting to thaw. Yet two things are still missing. One is coherence. Without a clearly articulated vision, co-ordinated action across a far wider range of policy risks being undermined. This report therefore attempts to set out a comprehensive template – one that is both holistic in its analysis and solutions, and global in its outlook. The second is leadership. The political climate is changing: the Liberal Democrats have consistently campaigned for more sensible legislation and the Conservatives have hinted at overhauling their approach to drugs as a key symbol of coming to terms with the modern world. For Labour the fact that the government's tough stance on crime is widely recognised creates space for a more nuanced approach to drugs. For these reasons, and given the weight of evidence that has now accrued on the damage of existing policies, the government would be foolish not to act. It would be a major blot on its copybook if in five or ten years' time, the scale of problem use had continued to soar and Britain had become increasingly out of step with its neighbours. Yet too many senior Labour politicians would still do almost anything rather than talk openly about drugs.

Case study: Nai Zindagi

Pakistan's drug problem has worsened considerably over the last ten years, in large measure as a side effect of events in Afghanistan. Latterly, the increase in refugees from the Taliban regime, and the ensuing concentration of poverty and poor infrastructure within Pakistan's borders, have contributed to the consolidation of local drug markets.

Today, one and a half million Pakistanis are chronic heroin users. Along with Britain, Pakistan now ranks among the world's top five consumer nations. The depth of the crisis and the pace of change are daunting. Yet, Nai Zindagi, a drug project working in Lahore, Islamabad, Quetta, Rawalpindi and Peshawar since 1990, has instead used them as a stimulus for turning conventional wisdom on its head and creating an impressive new approach to drugs.

In the beginning, Nai Zindagi offered only traditional treatment, albeit with a clear ethos of respect for its clients. While this was popular with clients used to local lock-downs whereby doctors achieved abstinence with their clients only because they chained them to their beds, it quickly became apparent it wasn't sustainable. Founder and director Tariq Zafar was faced with a cohort of treatment graduates reluctant to leave because they had nothing else to progress to. He wanted to work with highly marginalised drug users, yet treatment was expensive and public funding unpredictable. Besides, there was a dearth of trained counsellors to support the model.

But what began to trouble Tariq most were the assumptions underlying conventional ways of looking at the drug problem. Increasingly he felt they ascribed too much power to the substances people used, and denied individuals' own capacity to change. Funders' and policy makers' insistence on the goal of a drug free world seemed increasingly out of step with the challenges his clients faced – as was the specialised language and practice of the treatment world.

He drew on his previous commercial experience – which included co-ordinating Canon's local sales and importing agricultural technology to Pakistan – to begin adding vocational training and job creation to the range of initiatives offered by Nai Zindagi. Some clients introduced trades to Nai Zindagi; others set up treatment agencies of their own to increase coverage. Growth has been rapid, but the quality of therapeutic relationships has been maintained by keeping each initiative relatively small and linking them together under the overarching auspices of the Nai Zindagi management team.

Today, Nai Zindagi is the Diageo of the Forum projects, running seven businesses in and around Islamabad and Lahore, all of which employ around 80 per cent current or former drug users. In the Blue Quarter, Islamabad's smart commercial district, it runs a shop promoting an upmarket interior design service and marketing a distinctive line in environmentally friendly housing which is built to order. A concession selling middle market designer clothing in Lahore's glitzy Avari Hotel is one outlet for its smart handbags and travel wallets. Out of town, the project's mechanics buy old army jeeps, recondition them, road test and sell them on to NGOs and four wheel drive enthusiasts.

Underpinning the businesses are treatment services (detox and residential rehab) and feeding into these are extensive outreach services including street based needle and syringe exchanges, health promotion, counselling and advice. Drug users are also in the majority on the staff of these services, and all fully trained staff are paid similar rates to the project's doctors.

The project is determinedly oriented towards street users, around 8,000 of whom have access to health promotion, 1,200 to detox, 600 to rehab, 250 to vocational skills training and paid work every year. The numbers are small – and like all the projects profiled in this report, Nai Zindagi is not a panacea. But it does demonstrate the potential for models which both deal with the symptoms of drugs and their causes to produce durable outcomes.

As well as providing the structures by which clients can become independent, Nai Zindagi itself is largely autonomous. Its commercial activities return a profit of 30-35 per cent and at a stage when the programme was smaller paid for 70 per cent of its treatment costs – the project did not draw on donor funding for its core activities for two years.

Why it works

Honesty about drugs has been a critical starting point for Nai Zindagi. The project has found it easier than many to act pragmatically, attending to all its clients' problems of which the effects of drugs are only one aspect. It describes its job as enabling people to train their drug use, not deny it, and around 10 per cent of employees continue to use drugs in a functional way.

Through enterprise, Nai Zindagi supports clients as they engage with day to day life, its rewards and disappointments, risks and uncertainties, as well as opportunities. Clients earn salaries only when their skills are good enough. They learn the discipline that paying customers demand – for example, engineers working on the jeeps conduct numerous tests before passing the vehicles fit for sale. They learn how to anticipate problems and plan alternatives – and crucially, seek help as soon as they need it. In contrast, most drug agencies in the UK still work within a caring paradigm which, by Nai Zindagi's critique, replaces one dependency with another.

Innovation and openness about failure have been key to Nai Zindagi's and its clients' development. The failure of its early treatment services to promote long-term change is central to the Nai Zindagi story. So too are the mistakes of the first experiments with income generation; training began with no quality assurance and no market analysis or sales strategy – it came to an abrupt stop shortly after. But a willingness to learn from mistakes and draw lessons wherever they come from, combined with an appetite for attempting the unthinkable has strengthened the organisation's capacity to raise the stakes and reap greater rewards.

A fourth vital ingredient has been charismatic leadership – commercial, political and ethical. Managers of drug projects in the UK have often worked their way up from being involved in direct service provision.That can mean a limited vision – and little sense of what could be achieved beyond treatment. Tariq's vision and expertise are far broader and they are informed by his own experience of being a street drug user.

3. Problem drug use and the link with deprivation

Drug use is not new. Until 1860, all drugs were legal and many were in common use across the UK. William Gladstone and Florence Nightingale both used opium; Queen Victoria used cannabis. But throughout the twentieth century the evidence suggests that drug use has risen dramatically. When cocaine was criminalised, global production was around ten tonnes a year. Today 700 tonnes are produced annually. Illegal drugs now account for 8 per cent of global trade and represent the third largest industry in the world after oil and arms.

A BBC source suggests the number of illicit drug users in Britain has risen from around one million in the Sixties, to around 3 million in the Eighties, and to around 10 million now. The largest ever cohort of 20 to 24 year-olds (58 per cent) now report having used illicit substances at some point in their lives. Of 16 to 29 year-olds, a fraction under half (49 per cent) have used drugs, compared with only 28 per cent among their parents' generation of 30 to 59 year-olds; 16 per cent of this younger group use regularly compared with 3 per cent of the older group. The European Survey Project on Alcohol and other Drugs (ESPAD) found that there was an increase among 15 and 16 year-olds in the UK of heroin use from 1.6 per cent in 1995 to 2.7 per cent in 1999, and cocaine use from 2.6 per cent to 3.2 per cent over the same period. The proportion of 11 to 15 year-olds taking drugs consistently shows a small but steady increase and went up from 11 to 14 per cent between 1998 and 2002.

Much of this has been recreational use and is partly explicable as a consequence of changing values, and not in itself a major problem for Western societies. Despite media scares recreational use is generally manageable and fits within a lifestyle of clubbing and friendship networks which usually prevent overindulgence.

However, far sharper rises have occurred in problematic use, use that harms both the individual and the community of which they are a part.

By all indicators this misuse is now worsening rapidly. The number of people seeking help for their drug use has risen by 70 per cent over the last four years, and reflecting capacity in the treatment field, these figures possibly only represent the tip of the iceberg. The Office for National Statistics recorded a rise in heroin or morphine related deaths of 110 per cent between 1995 and 2000, up from 357 to 754. Cocaine deaths quadrupled over the same period, rising from 19 to 87 a year (again both sets of data are thought to under-represent the true figures). The figures also indicated a rise in the mixing of drugs, with over half the deaths linked to ecstasy, cocaine and amphetamines involving the use of other drugs. These figures are in many ways more telling than the much touted data on seizures. They point to a deepening crisis which existing approaches are failing to tackle.

The problem should be kept in perspective – many more deaths are attributable each year to alcohol and tobacco than to illicit drugs. One in three adults smokes tobacco, a cause of 120,000 premature deaths in Britain every year. But the side effects of drug misuse on lives and communities tend to be far more extreme and concentrated.

How should we understand the rise of drug misuse? And what should the answer be? In the media it is not hard to find many pet solutions: tougher penalties and life imprisonment for dealers on the one hand, legalisation on the other. For government the main priorities have been enforcement, which soaks up 62 per cent of the budget, managing international supply which accounts for 13 per cent, treatment and rehabilitation which account for 13 per cent, and prevention and education which take up the remaining 12 per cent.

There may be good reasons for this pattern of spending. However it does not reflect any rigorous analysis of the roots of the problem, or of what is likely to work in making a sustainable difference. The key issue is not availability or widespread drug use per se, but rather the pattern of drug use caused by, and in turn deepening, social exclusion. Any credible and effective solutions need to address these causes if they are to have a chance of success.

The causes of problem use

People take drugs for many reasons: pleasure, pain, fear, or because their friends do. And people from all backgrounds and classes misuse drugs, become addicted and in the worst cases wreck their lives.

But the pattern of who becomes addicted and who encounters problems is not random. Instead it shows a close link between drug misuse and social exclusion.

The first signs of this link became apparent in the US as some of the big cities encountered the first shocks of deindustrialisation. Previously the academic study of drug use had used traditional clinical research tools, focusing on individuals. The pioneering work done by the Chicago School of Sociology took a very different approach. In a series of studies in the postwar decades they looked at the clustering effect of linked, multiple problems. Their work showed clearly that poverty and decay in inner cities – not permissiveness, the influence of the media or any of the other factors sometimes cited – were the key causes of the heroin epidemics of the 1950s and 1960s in New York, Chicago and other US cities. In the 1980s the same factors helped to fuel the crack epidemics.

More recently a similar pattern has been seen in the UK. During the 1980s poverty increased and social exclusion became significantly worse in the UK. Between 1982 and 1996, the proportion of the population with incomes less than half the national average rose from 10 to 19 per cent. The United Nations Development Program (UNDP) showed that the poorest fifth in Britain had less spending power than their equivalents in other major Western countries, even than the US, and the Family Expenditure Survey recently revealed that the poorest households are paying a greater proportion of income in tax than the richest, partly because of tobacco duty, which represents 4.9 per cent of disposable income of the poorest fifth of households, compared to only 0.5 per cent for the richest fifth.

Studies of the 1980s heroin epidemics in Merseyside, Glasgow, Nottingham and South East London pointed to close correlations between the decay of the urban economy and community on the one hand, and rising drug misuse on the other.

The links between poverty and drug misuse in the UK

Twenty years of evidence of links has steadily accumulated. These are some of the key findings:

One study in the Wirral in the mid-1980s showed average prevalence of heroin users across the peninsular was 18.2 per 1,000 among 16-24 year-olds. But the spread ranged in different districts from nought to 162. The variation in geographical prevalence was highly correlated with seven indicators of background deprivation levels in each area (the correlation with treatment uptake among young people is shown in brackets): unemployment rate (.72), council tenancies (.67), overcrowding (.62), larger families (.49), unskilled employment (.39), single parent families (.69) and lack of access to a car (.58). All correlations reached statistical significance.

An analysis of 775 deaths from volatile substance abuse (VSA) in England, Scotland and Wales between 1985 and 1991, which set them against an ecological composite measure of deprivation (the Townsend index) showed that areas where a VSA death had occurred scored an average of 2.8 on the Townsend index, compared with an average score of .2 for those areas where a death hadn't occurred.

A study by Dr Laurence Gruer of some 3,715 drug-related emergency hospital admissions in Greater Glasgow from 1991 to 1996 plotted them by postcode using a standard index of deprivation. The admission rate from the most deprived areas exceeded that from the least deprived areas by a factor of 30, so that if the admission rate for the least deprived area had applied across the city, the number of admissions would have been 92 per cent lower. The authors noted that the relationship between deprivation and drug misuse is higher than any other health variable they had studied. This data is interesting because it also shows that relatively small reductions in deprivation hold the potential for significant health gains and harm reduction. Moving up from the most deprived to the second most deprived group reduced admissions by a factor of more than three.

An analysis of the 1995 Office of Population and Census Statistics Psychiatric Morbidity Survey presents one of the few pieces of research on the relationship between drug misuse and deprivation underpinned by a comprehensive national data set. Restricted to subjects aged 15-35, individuals were categorised according to:

- their degree of dependence (nought to four) on all illicit drugs based on intensity of use, sensed need, inability to cut down, tolerance and withdrawal symptoms;

- their degree of individual, as opposed to generalised area-wide profile, deprivation measured by unemployment, living in rented accommodation, not having use of a car, manual work status.

The likelihood of incurring a one to four score on the dependence scale increased in step with increases in the personal deprivation score. A person with extreme (four-point) deprivation was ten times more likely to have a positive dependence score than an individual with a zero deprivation score.

Patterns of this kind continue to show up today: for example a recent *Observer* survey showed that more than twice as many unemployed respondents (27 per cent) had ever used hard drugs than the average (12 per cent). The National Crime Survey shows that hard drug use is now seven times more prevalent among the unemployed than the employed or those not in receipt of benefits. The Social Exclusion Unit has found that of 16 to 18 year-olds not in education, training or work, 71 per cent report using drugs, compared with 47 per cent of their peers. School truants are twice as likely to have tried solvents and three times more likely to have tried drugs than those who don't truant. And the same patterns can be found in relation to different drugs and different countries: for example a study of cocaine and opiate overdose deaths in New York City in 1990-92 led the authors to suggest that poverty accounted for 69 per cent of the variance in mortality rates.

More recently, around a quarter of initial participants in the Progress initiative launched by the UK government to help drug users back into work, turned out to be off-register – neither claiming benefits nor earning income. Around 15 per cent were in receipt of incapacity benefit, and only five per cent received a training allowance. 50 per cent had not had a job during the past two years and a handful had never worked.

Health and deprivation
Although these findings are often ignored by policy-makers this data is not entirely surprising. There is a solid body of research on the links between relative deprivation and other forms of stress – depression, mental ill health, increased heart disease, suicide, crime, abuse and violence, other social ills.

There is also solid evidence on how the quality of the environment affects health and behaviour. According to recent research by Barnardo's, a child growing up at the least advantaged end of the socio-economic spectrum is twice as likely to die by the age of 15 as a more advantaged child. For men and women aged 15-29, suicide rates are approximately twice as high in deprived areas as they are in affluent areas. Unskilled men in the UK now have an overall, age-adjusted mortality rate three times that of professional men; the differential was only two-fold in the 1970s. The British Crime Survey (BCS) consistently shows that people who live in the poorest areas are most likely to be the victims of crime.

Lines of causation

The links between poverty and drug misuse are undeniable. But the nature of these links is not simple. Poverty does not directly cause addiction. Instead it increases the propensity to misuse – it weakens what are sometimes called the protective factors and it strengthens the risk factors. So even though the causes of deprivation are social, they are experienced individually.

Not everyone in a poor neighbourhood will become drug dependent, and those who do have their own set of reasons for responding to their circumstances within a particular idiom. But nevertheless the propensity to misuse is higher.

The complexity of the links between social factors and drug use can be confusing. For example an analysis of the BCS in 1996 led the researchers to conclude that urban areas populated by "professional people who tend to have active and varied leisure lives" have higher levels of illicit drug use by any age group, than even the most deprived areas. Part of the reason is that the BCS classifies drug use by all illicit drugs used 'ever' and 'in the past 12 months', i.e. it doesn't make the distinction between intensity, quantity or frequency of use.

Similarly lifetime use of drugs does not show any particular correlation with specific socio-economic conditions. However, all the more worrying aspects of drug use – age of first use, dependence, intravenous and risky use, health and social complications due to use, criminal involvement – are clearly linked to deprivation.

Just as people living with deprivation are at greater risk, they are also less likely to benefit from the things which might help them. Studies by Stimson and Blumberg of heroin users taking up treatment, showed that their socio-economic profile didn't differ from that of the wider population. Yet when analysts looked at access to care they found that it was closely correlated with socio-economic status – one example among many of the protective impact of effective public services (health inequalities in infants for example have been shown to be buffered during the school years, and to re-emerge along class lines after school).

These complexities are also apparent in relation to cigarettes and alcohol. Whereas in the past smoking was not correlated with class, today it is rising fastest among poor women, while alcohol misuse is rising amongst the middle classes. The key point is that this is a moving picture, in which one era's conventional wisdom can soon become out of date.

An holistic view

What follows from this brief overview of the evidence? The main message of the data is that we are seeing a process that is simultaneously social and economic, cultural and medical. To a medical specialist the problems are ones of addiction, to an economist the problems are ones of poverty and unemployment, and to an anthropologist they are problems that arise because in the face of devastated local economies, drug markets and street life provide alternative social networks by which users can regain a sense of identity, respect, recognition and authority.

In concluding its 1998 study of the impact of environment on drug use the government's Advisory Council on the Misuse of Drugs makes the point unequivocally: "We assert without any of the familiar hedging, that on strong balance of probability, deprivation is today, in Britain, likely often to make a significant causal contribution to the cause, complications and intractability of damaging kinds of drug misuse...Under such circumstances, local efforts to curb drug misuse are likely to be severely handicapped unless supported by wider schemes of urban regeneration, access to jobs and training, and other initiatives to combat social exclusion."

An holistic perspective is the most important starting point for any strategy to tackle drug misuse, which explains the relevance of the Asian projects profiled through this report to a UK setting. Better treatment that focuses on individuals rather than social causes, and policing solutions that deal with the symptoms, both at the heart of the government strategy, may help. But they are unlikely to stem the problem at its roots. Looking ahead they risk becoming even less effective, since many of the childhood traumas shaping future drug abuse have already happened.

For all this, UK policy is still based on the implicit assumption that law enforcement offers the best solution to the drug problem. Whatever shifts have been made in favour of prevention and treatment, they are relative and continue to take place within a legal framework which punishes users without adequately tackling dealers. Much of the rest of the world continues to take a similar view, still fundamentally influenced by the US policy-makers.

Yet even in the US there are signs of the tide turning. The Governor of New Mexico has proposed the decriminalisation of cannabis for personal use, without any damage to his popularity. The Republican New York governor George Pataki recently put before the New York legislature a bill to overturn the Rockefeller code, a draconian set of laws passed in 1973 bringing mandatory sentences of between 15 years and life for more serious drug offences and prison sentences for lesser ones which don't involve violence. The bill would affect current inmates, making some 500 of the 600 serving sentences over 15 years eligible for release.

Why the climate is changing
What is changing the climate for drug policy internationally?

One of the factors is economics. The American Centre on Addiction and Substance Abuse published a report last year calculating that US states spend an average of 13 per cent of their total budgets mopping up the fallout from drug abuse – more than they spend on higher education and ten times what they spend on prevention and treatment. Meanwhile, the Rand Corporation, like the NTORS study in the UK, demonstrated the cost effectiveness of demand reduction, that every dollar spent on treatment saved seven on additional drug related services. Add to this the loss of income through taxation – on a UK heroin market currently estimated to be worth £4.5bn – and the argument becomes compelling.

A second factor is public opinion. Almost half the British public believes cannabis should not be illegal and 99 per cent think it should have the lowest policing priority. Yet 90 per cent of all offences are for possession, of which 75 per cent, or 90,000, are for cannabis and there are huge variations in the issuing of police cautions – from 22 to 72 per cent of all cases depending on the force.

A third is the emergence of a more holistic approach to crime. A fifth of all people arrested in Britain are on heroin. A recent study showed that 700 career heroin users committed 70,000 crimes within a three month period to fund their habit. The researchers believe the average heroin dependent steals goods worth £43,000 every year. One response is to call for more ferocious policing – but many police have come to the conclusion that long-term it will be more effective to deal with the causes.

A fourth is a growing sense of despair at the failure of policy. To take just one measure: heroin-related deaths per million population across Europe rose by 150 per cent between 1995 and 1999. Of the total 9,373 drug related deaths in the UK during 1999, 3,000 were recorded by coroners as accidental and 3,800 as either suicide or undetermined, reflecting both the unwanted risks and severe alienation and despair accompanying heavy drug use.

A fifth and final reason is international experience which is showing an increasing plurality of approaches. Dutch decriminalisation of cannabis has successfully segregated the market such that, despite some problems of 'drugs tourism', heroin use in Holland has remained stable where in the UK, Norway, Italy and Belgium among others have all seen dramatic and continuing increases under prohibition.

Case study: Mukti Sadan

Mumbai in India is one of the world's greatest cities. But away from the business districts, smart nightclubs and glossy shop fronts lies that all too familiar corollary to rapid urbanisation – some of the world's largest and most notorious slums, with poor sanitation, underemployment and despair. The prospect of the good life for the majority of slum dwellers remains as illusory as the fictions concocted in nearby Bollywood. Instead, for many, heroin has come to offer an increasingly attractive alternative. Since 1989, this is where Mukti Sadan has developed a fresh approach to drugs.

What it is?
Mukti Sadan is a broad based community programme driven by its commitment to servicing drug users – 1,200 of them at any one time. The project allows chaotic street users to access help informally through night shelters for prostitutes, temporary detox camps set up in the midst of the slums and drop-in advice centres. Outreach teams distribute clean needles and medication and counsel families so that they can care for family members whose struggles with drug use can at times seem perpetual and overwhelming. Drug users can stabilise their problems with the help of medication, structured social support and general health services. They can learn new skills through workshops and training schemes and renew their contacts beyond drug-using circles.

The breadth of social networks encouraged by the project sets it apart from most drug services in the UK. Women from the wider community work in the screen-printing workshops, and their children attend the project's school. Young people at risk of entrenched drug use benefit from dedicated vocational programmes which help them take steps towards viable alternatives to employment in drug markets.

The other major distinguishing feature is Mukti Sadan's employment and wealth creating portfolio. Recognising the role of work in maintaining people's involvement in mainstream communities, the project has begun training graduates of its drug treatment services in how to run microbusinesses. In fields such as rag recycling, serving hot food or henna painting, these businesses are unlikely ever to grow very large, but they are enough to support a household and present a viable form of enterprise where access to capital is poor and the market modest. Through the project, clients can also access much needed credit and business advice.

Three years ago, Mukti Sadan embarked on its most ambitious employment initiative so far: exploiting its contacts in industry and access to commercial expertise, it bought a machine tool workshop, negotiated sub-contracts to supply small parts for manufacturers of industrial equipment and set about training drug users more systematically. Drug users must first learn a series of technical skills – how to file, lathe and polish metal components. If they successfully complete their initial training, they may undertake a paid apprenticeship where they work more independently and earn a rudimentary salary the equivalent to that of a shop worker or junior government clerk. On completion, they apply for jobs in the workshop or receive help securing paid work elsewhere in the city. In a small way Mukti Sadan acts like a recruitment agency. Daily on-site assessments, medication, counselling and self-help groups ensure clients make steady progress safely.

What it achieves
Outcomes from the tool shop are comparable to those of the mainstream New Deal programmes in the UK. So despite the fact the client group has far greater 'distance to travel' between the street and work, of the first 51 recruits to the tool shop, 23 have found work, while 8 are still training. During the past two years, around 15 small businesses have been established with Mukti Sadan's support.

Though relapse is still common, rates are lower than the figure of more than nine in ten in the UK. Around twenty per cent of clients entering treatment become stable, while a further 56 per cent become moderately stable – able to begin the process of retraining and rebuilding their lives.

Why it works
Mukti Sadan works with whole communities rather than attempting to meet an ever-increasing demand for services from isolated sub-cultures within them. Staff are taught to broker relationships and make deals

around resources, and of investments human, social and cultural, as well as to act as advocates and service providers. They mobilise families and the faith communities, Christian, Muslim and Hindu, and traditional healers, to work with drug users.

The project has been rigorous about experimenting and building on what works in cycles of action research and highly reflective practice. For example, staff quickly identified that support from women outside the drug-using groups was crucial because as 'moral guardians' of their families, they often determined who was in and who was out and how informal resources were allocated. Although these women were initially very sceptical about the project's mission, the creation of a school to benefit their children helped to convince them to get involved and take part in the project's workshops for themselves.

The project has attracted a sufficiently diverse staff team to enable drug users to move from dependency to work. Though the founder and director Shobha Kapoor, trained in social work and cut her teeth running the first hospital-based drug unit in India, she has had the foresight to recruit tutors, engineers, marketing specialists and entrepreneurs, as well as the more usual doctors and community workers.

4. The limitations of current approaches

New problems, old solutions

While the context of drug supply and demand has been dramatically transformed, drug policy has remained stubbornly anachronistic. Along with the US, the UK has long pursued a twin track approach to drug policy that combines prohibition with treatment. Labour's 1998 National Anti-Drug Strategy promoted a 'balanced approach' and promised a new direction, but essentially did little more than shift the balance of spending. Whereas under the Conservatives, around three quarters of the drug budget was invested in law enforcement, and a quarter in treatment with waiting lists of up to a year as a result, Labour has set out to change the balance so that by 2003 only 55 per cent of an expanded budget will be spent on policing and intelligence.

The weakness of this shift is that in real terms it represents a greater spend on both prohibition (which doesn't appear to work) and treatment (which works only poorly in isolation), and offers no answers to the deeper causes. At first glance it seems unlikely to achieve much in relation to the underlying trends in drug use and availability (see Figures 1 and 2). This chapter therefore addresses in more detail what works and what doesn't in the current policy mix.

The fallout from prohibition

Many states have tried to prohibit drugs. Not all have had quite such a disastrous experience as the US prohibition of alcohol in the 1920s, which left behind a rudely healthy system of organised crime. But none can claim to have succeeded by any simple criteria.

Few make any sustained difference in availability. Even highly targeted policing can fail – a recent simultaneous crackdown on over two

Figure 1: Traditional drug treatment fails to curb exponential growth in the numbers experiencing problem use

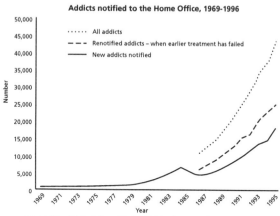

Addicts notified to the Home Office, 1969-1996

...... All addicts

– – – Renotified addicts – when earlier treatment has failed

——— New addicts notified

Source: Addicts notified to the Home Office 1969-1996. Data from Home Office Statistical Bulletin.
Published in Drugs: Dilemma and choices, The Royal College of Psychiatrists, 2000.

Figure 2: Rising seizures – alongside greater availability*

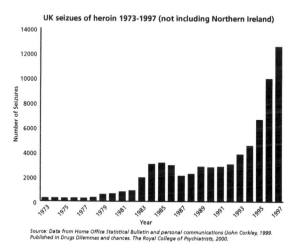

UK seizues of heroin 1973-1997 (not including Northern Ireland)

Source: Data from Home Office Statistical Bulletin and personal communications (John Corkley, 1999.
Published in Drugs Dilemmas and chances. The Royal College of Psychiatrists, 2000.

* Research has shown the weight of seizures to be a consistent indicator of the real level of supply – it is reckoned that ten
kilos of heroin hit the streets for every one kilo seized.

hundred known dealers in London, the largest ever in the UK, made no perceptible dent in a resilient market.

Most have been hugely costly relative to their successes: the US war on drugs has cost literally hundreds of billions of dollars. In the UK a single prosecution for cannabis possession typically costs well over £10,000.

Some have simply displaced the problem. Bolivia and Peru for example successfully curbed coca production only for it to move to neighbouring Colombia, along with an influx of illegal immigrants following new sources of work.

Some have amplified social divisions. In the US, young black men are far more likely than their white counterparts to be imprisoned as a result of drug possession. In the UK, The Prison Reform Trust points out that 2 in 5 of all female prisoners are jailed for drug offences compared to 1 in 14 men.

Some have institutionalised hypocrisy: leading figures in some Latin American governments were able to accept US aid for the war on drugs while also privately profiting from it. Morocco officially bans cannabis, yet forcing militant farmers to abandon cultivation and see their annual incomes fall to subsistence levels is politically risky. The country remains the source of 80 per cent of Europe's supply. During 2000 the Taliban declared a policy of prohibition while secretly taking a cut from the still substantial trade. Closer to home, officers from the National Crime Squad have been arrested for the possession and supply of drugs.

Others have solved one problem only to create another. The level of disproportionate violence exacted against farmers of coca leaf in Colombia is now well publicised, but less well known are the health problems among their families (chemical burns and respiratory difficulties) and the environmental degradation that are a direct result of indiscriminate crop spraying. Malaysia has all but eradicated the use of hard drugs through draconian laws for even small possession charges. However, it has done so by incarcerating large numbers of users. Subsequently Malaysians have largely swapped smoking heroin for injecting as supplies have became scarce, and HIV infection rates have soared. A similar pattern occurred in northern Thailand during the early 1990s as a direct result of UN crop eradication initiatives.

Still others have missed the point. So much of the drugs industry takes place behind closed doors that formal policing is only ever likely to address the tip of the iceberg: one study in Glasgow showed that 60 per cent of young people who had used drugs scored from older siblings or were given drugs by their parents. Ethnographic studies from North America show that zero tolerance policies for street drug dealing only temporarily hold local markets in check and can have unplanned and highly undesirable side effects such as an increase in the involvement of children who attract less scrutiny. New Deal for Community managers working in some of the poorest areas of Britain give anecdotal accounts of similar consequences.

Prohibition has certainly created a thriving industry of its own, but it has flatly failed to address the original problem it set out to curb. Instead it has concentrated efforts on easy targets such as small time user-dealers, poor farmers, and seizures of soft drugs. And by giving the illusion of success (arrests and seizures have long shown substantial increases year on year) while basically preserving the status quo, it is likely they have played an unhealthy role in creating the conditions for rapid sustained growth. Sized at around US $100 bn, the drug industry is in economic terms a huge success story, a vast global industry that accounts for as much as half of some countries' income. But untaxed and unregulated a lucrative platform for a range of other criminal interests from sex to arm trade.

Recent diversification into more stringent financial controls promises to bolster traditional policing by making it more difficult for drug barons to trade conventionally. There is no doubt international co-operation to shut down opportunities for money laundering, root out banking transactions that are propping up illegal activity and more effectively seize drug barons' assets could all substantially help to increase the costs of selling drugs and will focus attention on the orchestrators at the top of the supply chain.

But past experience tells us that the law of supply and demand means that disrupting distribution may well drive up street prices, thereby having the opposite effect to that intended, by simply improving the rewards for those who can do business. Like past attempts at disruption the impact of this round may at best be temporary and may even further develop the industry's capacity to innovate.

Where the law is working

Experience of prohibition isn't the only counterintuitive lesson that drug policy-makers have been slow to learn. Those countries like Holland that have decriminalised cannabis have succeeded in segregating the market between hard and soft drugs. In contrast to the UK which has some of the toughest laws in Europe and the highest rates of addiction, Holland has seen its use of heroin stabilise. Puncturing the appeal of drug taking has also paid dividends on other fronts: while a fraction under half (49 per cent) of British 15 year-olds have tried cannabis, only a fifth of their Dutch peers have done so. In other words the law has an important role in conveying societal norms, but not the one we traditionally ascribe it.

Dampening demand for drugs

As law enforcement has failed to deliver on its promises, demand reduction has increasingly come to be seen as the best, and most humane, solution to the problem of drugs. Whereas supply reduction depends on dealing with long chains of criminal activity, far beyond the reach of law enforcement agencies, the children and young people at risk of becoming drug users are close at hand, and can be reached through their families, schools and communities. Just as important, those people who do use illicit drugs often at some point face up to the damage they are doing to themselves and welcome the support of services designed to help them cut their consumption.

The case for demand reduction has been easy to make because some of its tools – drug education and treatment for drug users encountering difficulties – are relatively uncontroversial. For decades their advocates have provided a rare voice of reason in a field full of ferocious passions and prejudices.

Yet on closer inspection the evidence for effectiveness turns out to be much weaker than one might hope. Drug education is a good example. A recent, and typical, study by the Drugs Prevention Advisory Service (DPAS) showed that although 41 per cent of 14 to 16 year-olds said they were less likely to take drugs after participating in a drug education course, the one year follow-up showed that there had been no change in their actual use of drugs. There are other arguments for drug education such as helping people to use drugs in a more informed way, but the case for spending large sums of money on it to reduce demand is unproven.

Similar doubts apply to drug treatment. Although the UK government will have doubled investment in treatment by the end of its second term, the evidence on the effectiveness of treatment is much more complex, and ambiguous, than its advocates claim.

What treatment does achieve

The good news for treatment advocates is that the largest ever longitudinal study of the impact of drug treatment on problematic use in the UK, the National Treatment Outcome Research Study (NTORS) has since the mid-1990s confirmed what a litany of smaller studies have shown over the years – that on balance, and subject to the caveats, treatment does work. When carried out well, it:

• Reduces the use of illicit drugs – thereby preserving household expenditure for essentials and dampening local drug markets;

- Improves physical health – users have better liver functioning, fewer venal infections, abscesses etc. One recent Swiss study went as far as to suggest that 12 per cent of heroin dependents die if rejected from treatment, compared with one per cent in treatment;

- Leads to improved mental and emotional health – the proportion of those who have recently contemplated suicide halves after two years in contact with treatment agencies;

- Cuts crime – every extra £1 spent on treatment contributes to a cost saving of £3 from crime, although other studies remind us that persistent offenders do not automatically curtail their offending without specific measures and many drug users commit no other crime than that of consuming illicit substances.

There are problems with selection: around a third of clients drop out of treatment near the beginning of their episode because they are judged not to be making sufficient progress, leaving only those who already show high levels of motivation and self-control to benefit from professionals' attentions. But clearly, these are significant gains, and they have been achieved in humane ways, going a long way to respecting the human rights of those involved. If anyone remains in any doubt as to the legitimacy of their arguments, they need look no further than the HIV epidemic that never happened in the UK. In the mid-1980s, injecting drug users looked set to be a prime constituency of the forecast epidemic. Thanks in part to the then highly controversial efforts of the harm reduction wing of treatment professionals, the rapid establishment of needle and syringe exchanges ensured the disease never became predominant among this group in the UK, in striking contrast to East and Central European countries which have as a result suffered a hugely greater death-toll.

Why treatment is a partial solution
However, the case for education and treatment is much less robust than it's advocates claim. Their analysis of why people become addicted is

flawed and their methods are at best partially successful (see Figure 3). On their own, these methods risk dealing with symptoms rather than causes; at worst, a big expansion of treatment could simply create a bigger revolving door for drug users rather than a lasting solution.

Figure 3: The limitations of treatment

Treatment approaches	Health promotion, drug education, needle and syringe exchanges, advice and information services.	Substitute prescribing, counselling, residential rehabilitation, '12 Steps' self-help and detoxification.	Outreach, dual diagnosis and interagency work.
Limitations	Supply knowledge and technical equipment, but do not improve unhealthy environments. Fail to set up credible sanctions and rewards to motivate change. Those who are worst off are least likely to benefit.	Treat problems symptomatically – high relapse rates once support is removed. By being apolitical, do not alleviate the substantive burdens their clients face. Rigid rules exclude the heaviest users at the point of entry.	Without purchasing power, lack leverage. Reflect weaknesses in local structures and priorities.

The treatment industry (see Annex for further detail on orthodox drug treatment approaches) has a view of how drugs work that has taken shape over the last century as the physiology of habitual drug use has gripped observers as much as it has preoccupied its subjects. Every child grows up learning that 'hard' drugs exert a powerful effect on our bodies and minds and that before very long, their influence becomes overwhelming. Many substance use specialists take a similar view. They believe that if the body's biochemistry can be manipulated to create a window of stability, an habitual drug user will cease craving the substances that cause them so much harm and change their behaviour to seek more constructive pursuits. This is the principle behind most methadone programmes and the prescription of other opiate alleviating medications such as buprenorphine. It also lies behind experiments with antagonists such as naloxone which block a substance's effect, the use of anti-depressants to relieve the crashing lows induced by heavy cocaine use, and the use of alternative therapies such as auricular acupuncture (in the ear) to stimulate the body's own endorphins.

The persistence of a biomedical understanding of addiction is understandable. People choose to use heroin, crack, cocaine, barbiturates and amphetamines, and also cigarettes, alcohol and prescription drugs, increasingly in polydrug cocktails, precisely because they transform the way they feel. A biomedical approach is also understandable for another reason: the effects of drug abuse, up to and including death, are best understood in biomedical terms.

It comes as a surprise to many, however, to discover that strictly biomedical conceptions of addiction have little explanatory power. They cannot explain, for example, why only around one per cent of people who use heroin or cocaine become dependent users. Or why the majority of people who begin using regularly wean themselves off their drug of choice when the costs outweigh the benefits. The biomedical model cannot explain why medical treatment programmes promote health savings, less infection, abscesses, depression but not further reaching changes in behaviour, why prison leavers who went straight inside make a hit the first thing they secure on the outside, or why methadone patients often increase the amount of alcohol they drink to unhealthy levels, or use heroin on top though they are experiencing no withdrawals. Nor can it account for why people will seek out the most unpromising alternatives when the usual drugs aren't available. A Cambodian member of the Forum network reports the injection of large quantities of vitamins and even snake poison among its clients; men in the Sahel are becoming increasingly dependent on sugar at the expense of their health and that of their wives and children.

The inadequacy of the model is most strikingly thrown into relief by the experience of the American Vietnam war veterans. Drawn from a reasonably representative cross section of the general public, a massive 70 per cent of them used heroin to deal with the pressures on the frontline. But far from creating a generation of opiate abusers, only 1 to 3 per cent continued to use on their return to civilian life, despite the absence of any targeted treatment – the same sort of proportion as the rest of the population.

To be fair, even the most committed clinician acknowledges that every individual with a problem drug habit has an intimate relationship with their addiction and that treatment can only be effective if the psychosocial context of consumption is taken into account. The best recognise that the behaviours an individual wraps round their drug use form a pattern which needs to be reshaped into an entirely new lifestyle if treatment is to work (and when a lay person judges someone to have an 'addictive personality', they are indicating what a pervasive influence the psychological and social investment in a particular pattern of behaviour can hold). To this end, a client's initial assessment, and later their regular reviews, will involve discussion of their home life, housing status, informal social support and sense of well-being and recommendations will be adjusted accordingly. Clients are unlikely to enter into a sustained treatment episode without at least the offer of brief counselling to help them adapt. But even those who take a very broad view of treatment, encompassing physiological change and psychological change, are still locked into a highly individualistic view of addiction, which simply ignores the social factors at work.

As a result we have witnessed a marked change in levels of problem drug use in the UK since the 1980s into which the treatment world has made few inroads.

The answer is not to do away with legislation and treatment. Both are part of the toolkit with which we can effectively manage drugs. But they must be framed by policies underpinned by a full analysis of the problem and allied to more holistic approaches that tackle all of the causes as well as the symptoms.

Case study: Sharan

Opium smoking has long been common in the slums of Delhi. But the use of illicit drugs didn't become a critical problem until the early 1990s when Delhi became linked into the new heroin distribution routes to the West. Heroin was by now cheaper than cannabis or home-brewed alcohol, and quickly won a large market. At the same time, faced with high levels of unemployment and underemployment, slum dwellers tended to be the most willing recruits to work in the new drug markets and were employed to take the greatest risks.

Soon many found that their drug habits had become uncontrollable. The unlucky ones were imprisoned, persecuted, contracted AIDs or were disowned by families ashamed of their behaviour. Others found their way onto the streets – indeed research suggests that 90 per cent of Delhi's drug users are homeless.

Drugs had become one of the defining problems for the slums. They both excited members of the community with the rare prospect of a decent income, and divided it as many were appalled by the fallout.

Sharan is an NGO that had been involved in development in Delhi, mobilising community groups to deal with health, education and regeneration at a grassroots level, for over thirty years. But it is the work it has developed with drug users during this period of rapid change that has attracted international attention.

Sharan runs a wide range of drug services – street based advice, needle and syringe exchanges, community detox camps, prescribing programmes using buprenorphine and latterly methadone, counselling, on-going support groups, wound dressing and other drug related primary care services, a newsletter and advocacy service. What is distinctive is the way they are linked up.

In most UK settings, clients will find only narrow services and a referral or gate-keeping system to join them up. By contrast Sharan tries to offer a more seamless service and a higher degree of continuity in relationships with staff. Abstinence and harm reduction services are on offer at different stages in a client's recovery and they are complemented by vocational training and access to income generation schemes and credit when stability has been achieved. The project has acknowledged that recovery is rarely a linear path with neat sequential steps. So rather than being run as bolt-ons at the end of treatment, work related initiatives are introduced as an integral part of it. As clients progress they can see the benefits – and the cost of relapse. If they do relapse, Sharan is flexible at moving clients to different treatment services. Like Mukti Sadan and Kaleidoscope, Sharan is closely tied into the community so drug users are more easily able to reconnect once their drug use is in check.

Where Sharan has probably been most enterprising is in the business-like approach it is has taken to meeting the new challenges faced by slum communities. Against a backdrop of widespread fatalism, inertia and hostility, it provided one of the first strategic responses to the rising tide of drugs and AIDs. The difficulties were immense. Prejudice against drug users was deep-felt – the official position ten years ago was that drug users should be left to die. Effective models of reducing harm and curtailing the spread of blood borne diseases could only work if there was sufficient coverage. Existing models such as health education, needle and syringe exchanges and substitute prescribing all needed to be allied to training, work and regeneration to make a durable and cost effective impact in highly marginalised settings.

Since there were no staff trained to work in this new context Sharan set about training drug users themselves to roll out the programme to greater numbers in Delhi. Creating a track record of success, the project attracted additional support and investment from European governments, the EU and UN agencies. Then it began to link up other Forum members in India (the Calcutta Samaritans, TTK in Madras, Sahara and Mukti Sadan) to train drug users to undertake local rapid assessments and replicate some of its approaches. It was instrumental in helping to join up like-minded projects to act corporately across Asia under the auspices of Forum and more recently, the Asian Harm Reduction Network.

What it achieves
The project is realistic – it recognises that small non-profit organisations cannot deal with the full scale of the problem. But it has demonstrated that drug users themselves can be part of the solution – they now make

up 80 per cent of the permanent staff, among them doctors, managers and general drug workers alike. It has also shown an unusual ability, delivering drug services to tens of thousands of people in five of India's major cities. Despite the difficulties, it has proven an effective critic of government apathy and a powerful advocate for change grounded in the day to day experience of what works. Under the visionary leadership of Luke Samson, it has formed an alliance of grassroots projects addressing their clients' problems in the round, they last year hosted the first International Harm Reduction Conference in Asia and played a key role in finally persuading the Indian government to put sustainable harm reduction at the heart of its policies.

Why it works
Sharan has developed a home-grown style of practical drug activism which offers several dividends. It creates jobs for drug users by rebuilding their confidence – not least through the example of staff who understand their experience; it helps the community through lower crime and fear and by challenging a sense of powerlessness and it has contributed to national and international policy debates by demonstrating good practice, not just talking about it.

5. Holistic demand reduction

So how can the demand for drugs be reduced? Common sense dictates that the answer must lie in dealing with all of the factors that produce demand in the first place. Surprisingly, however, much of what passes for drug policy has simply side-stepped rigorous analysis of the causes of demand for drugs, jumping instead to 'one club' solutions, based on one-cause analyses. The results are predictable: policies that continually fail by any objective measure.

This chapter sets out a crucial step towards a more successful policy: a more systematic map of the factors that lead people to become problem drug users, drawing on the experience of some of the projects profiled in this report.

The risk factors of problem drug use
A good starting point for understanding the various factors that feed drug misuse is the index developed by Eric Blakebrough through the work of Kaleidoscope, the only UK member and one of the founding projects of Forum (see Figure 4). The index describes the cluster of factors in a person's life that make them more vulnerable to problem drug use. Even when all are present, some people manage to resist drugs. But their presence means the odds of problem use rise significantly.

Contact with drugs
The first factor is access. Today most people have ready access to illicit drugs with minimal effort – indeed, they were probably the first product to adapt to the 24 hour society. The internet is providing new tools for marketing and sales, older siblings and other family members remain a flexible and popular source for younger consumers and friends are the suppliers for the vast majority of consumers. The Department for Trade and Industry anticipates that nanotechnology in the form of handheld gadgets will soon enable small, and therefore

hard to detect or divert, amounts of drugs to be produced at the point of sale. Some predict that domestically synthesised drugs will dominate future markets – meta-amphetamine is already the fastest growing drug in the US and belies the belief that drug production is only something that takes place in the hands of evil suppliers abroad.

However, as the evidence shows, although widespread and frequent contact means that it is now almost deviant among teenagers and young adults to abstain from using an illicit substance at some point, it does not alone account for entrenched use. Millions use drugs but they only become a problem for a far smaller group. Access is a necessary but not sufficient condition for problem use.

Lack of identification with the mainstream
The second factor helps to explain why some start on the path to misuse. People who feel cut off and excluded from mainstream society and culture tend to look for alternative means of self-expression and recognition; drug cultures provide a ready option. Many teenagers use drugs for a time in part for this reason. But only those with no alternative attach themselves to drug-related lifestyles long-term.

Ethnographic street studies have shown how "taking care of business" lends motivation, meaning and structure to a drug user's day even more than the drugs themselves. One study by Lofland also concluded that dealing affords the most "proximate and performable" way of generating income for the dispossessed and low skilled in times of high unemployment. And, as another study by Oetting and Beauvais shows, early drug use is explained less by traditional notions of peer pressure, than by the dynamics whereby peer clusters, "small, cohesive, marked by closely shared attitudes and beliefs", provide young people with a sense of acceptance and belonging.

Sense of alienation caused by bereavement or trauma
The third factor is past loss. A remarkably high proportion of dependent drug users experienced the death of, or severe physical or emotional

abuse from, a close intimate during their childhood. With the support of family, friends or trusted professionals, people can come to terms with their grief, anger and self-hatred. But for others the comfort of mind-altering substances is a desperately needed substitute for unconditional love and intimacy.

No suitable ally or pastime
The fourth factor is present loneliness. Friends, allies and companions can provide reward and recognition. Without them, it is all too easy to fill the vacuum with drugs. And once started, it can become ever harder to get out: as a rule the more time spent in heavy drug using circles, the greater the barriers – economic, social, cultural – to making connections with others. One of the reasons that many ex-users who have been through traditional treatment relapse and return to treatment is simply that they were too lonely and aimless; stripped of their drug-using friendship groups and the interest and advice of treatment staff, they have nothing else to fall back on.

A blocked future
The fifth factor is future hopelessness. Fatalism and short-termism can be rational responses to a lack of future prospects. Studies by the evolutionary psychologists Daly and Wilson demonstrate how homicide rates soar when young men in the physical and social ghettos of urban America feel trapped and powerless to improve their lives. Without hope for the future, all kinds of risk-taking behaviour increase.

The features of holistic rehabilitation
Together these five factors go a long way to explain both who becomes a dependent drug user, and why the numbers have risen so sharply in recent years.

Put simply the environmental causes of these five factors are all currently favourable in the UK: increasing availability because of the combination of abundant supply and effective distribution networks; alienation as the traditional bonds of family, community and work

Figure 4: What makes people vulnerable to problem drug use

The Kaleidoscope at–risk index of problem drug use

Contact	with drugs
Lack of identification	with the mainstream (through family, friends or peers)
Sense of alienation	caused by unresolved bereavement or trauma
No suitable ally or pastime	to provide emotional support and positive feedback
A blocked future	educational, employment and relationship opportunities inhibited

weaken; unstable and often abusive families; social exclusion and long-term unemployment in some communities.

Work in the criminal justice field has shown that long-term strategies for cutting crime have to begin by strengthening the protective factors at work in the lives of people at risk of getting involved in crime. Much the same applies to drug misuse. This in essence is the insight of the Forum projects which, in their very different ways, all attempt to deal with all the risk factors: changing people's lives rather than seeing drug use simply as a medical problem.

The following chapter sets out how Forum members address each of the key causes of problem drug use.

Case study: Sahara

Sahara has its headquarters in Delhi and complements its partner with more residential care, abstinence-based services and a greater emphasis on preventing and dealing with HIV and AIDs. Through its base in Manipur, one of the most inaccessible parts of north-east India on the border of Burma, it has first hand experience of picking up the casualties of aggressive drug supply and attempting to prevent people flocking to India's major cities in search of greater prospects.

What it is?
Sahara began as a service for people with HIV and AIDs in northern India, in Delhi, Pune, Mumbai and Manipur. The project's staff offered medical and social care through day centres, respite and residential programmes. They also looked after patients in government hospitals and trained families who didn't have access to other services to take care of patients in their homes.

Sahara's work changed gear during the late 1980s and 1990s. When it began it was assumed that AIDs sufferers would have little time to live and that the priority was to provide respite care. However, as patients responded to treatment, the project increasingly found itself called upon to provide a wider range of services. Because inevitably a high proportion of its clients were injecting drug users, Sahara increasingly built up services focused on drugs such as outreach and the street based distribution of needles and syringes, help and advice, counselling, detox, rehab and halfway houses to help people back into the community.

More recently, like the other Forum members, Sahara has started setting up businesses to train and pay its clients. It now runs a second-hand clothing store which has been a runaway success; small scale clothing manufacturing (run by a group of women who pool childcare and work from home); carpentry and woodwork manufacturing and selling; and screen-printing handling business cards, leaflets and annual reports.

With its roots in community development, Sahara has evolved differently from the other projects in this report. It has built capacity rapidly and at little cost because it has seen itself largely as a facilitator of community based action rather than a top-down service provider. It inspires in former clients a sense of vocation which is at once altruistic – many want to give something back to the communities they have come from – and self-serving – fulfilling a sense of service has proven a satisfying alternative to the streets. Its core services employ only ten full-time staff and overheads are kept at an economical US $80,000 a year. The large corps of former drug users it has mobilised are best thought of as professional volunteers (like, for example, The Samaritans in the UK and VSO overseas). While they take dividends of funds when the project is flush, in the main they work in return for food, subsistence, accommodation and high levels of camaraderie.

What it has achieved
Sahara now provides services for around 1,000 drug users every year and reaches 2,000 more, mainly HIV positive people in the community. Its businesses remain fairly small but they are breaking even ahead of their targets and look set to expand quickly.

Its greatest success has arguably been in changing attitudes in the medical profession. When Sahara's staff first went into hospitals, health professionals were scared of touching HIV and AIDs patients. They would hand out medication, but deprive patients of essential nursing given to others – they literally worked at arms' length. Unsurprisingly, patients failed to thrive. Sahara changed all that by deliberately making its hands-on care highly conspicuous. The hospitals changed their policies and patients' became more receptive to treatment. Sahara has challenged the fatalism among drug users in the slums in a similar way, choosing to send in former drug users trained in health promotion rather than just sharing more kind words.

Why it works
Like Kaleidoscope, one of the project's most striking features is a strong emphasis on hospitality and respect for clients. People are welcomed as if they were one of the family, rather than as recipients of a traditional service. So for example personal loans are often made to clients, to cover everything from rent arrears to purchasing equipment, safe in the knowledge that they will be repaid because the ethos of the project elicits a strong commitment from clients themselves. Food and facilities are shared, and help and support is available round the clock. The director, Neville Selhore, leads by example, living and sleeping at one of the Delhi based rehabs.

The other key is that by providing clients with structure and expertise, a small injection of resources and large amounts of encouragement, Sahara has succeeded in releasing drug users' confidence in developing their own response to problems holistically and sustainably. Acting together they have created a rich alternative to the streets which meets their needs personally, socially and economically.

6. Lessons from Asia

Why we should learn from Asia

In the drugs field as elsewhere policy-makers are far more likely to look to the US or Europe, than further afield. It tends to be assumed that less developed countries are so fundamentally different from the West in terms of their standards of living, institutions and attitudes, that there is little prospect of taking solutions from one environment to the other. Given the exciting developments now taking place in European drug policy the tendency for the West to look to its own solutions is probably if anything being reinforced.

But there are good reasons for taking a more global perspective. In many fields of social policy it is now recognised that the prosperous north can learn from the poorer south. Social exclusion and poverty are obviously very different in a city like Glasgow or Chicago than they are in Mumbai or Lahore. But some of the features are similar. This is why practical solutions like the Grameen Bank's approaches to microcredit have been successfully transplanted from the Bangladeshi countryside to the poor communities of north America and Europe.

Drug policy could soon become another field in which the West stops preaching and starts learning. Many of the causes of drug dependency are surprisingly similar, as are some of the solutions.

It would be wrong to present any of these models as panaceas. The evidence base remains thin; there are no holistic projects anywhere in the world which have been subjected to the full rigour of research. But the thirty or so projects that are now part of the Forum network are promising examples of a different, more rounded approach that fits what we know of the causes of drug dependency much better than the one-dimensional approaches so common in the West. And all show what drug policy might look like if it can evolve beyond the limitations of depending on legal prohibition on the one hand and medical treatment on the other.

Most have drawn not only on the expertise of health professionals but also on the experience of drug users themselves, the inspiration of faith communities, and the energy of entrepreneurs. Much more than in the West their work is understood as integral to development. And much more than in the West they have recognised that crisis demands constant innovation and willingness to question sacred cows.

Although they have faced scepticism and outright opposition as the full impact of drugs dependency has become more visible, and as the costs associated with AIDs and the role of drug use in spreading the epidemic have belatedly been acknowledged, even their critics have grudgingly recognised their contribution. The result is that over the last decade each of the projects described here, though different, has embedded the best of what the West has learnt about medical interventions into programmes which offer a far richer approach.

A comprehensive approach to risk

The key contribution of the Forum projects is to offer a direct answer to a proper analysis of causes. More than the projects to be found in Europe or North America what is distinctive about them is that they offer a comprehensive answer to all of the key risk factors associated with problem drug use.

To reduce contact

The first priority is to help remove people from direct access to drug markets, and put them into a context where drugs are the exception not the rule. In the UK this is done temporarily in residential retreats – but once the user returns to the outside it may be hard to avoid drugs. In the Asian projects, by contrast, the aim has been to create long-term alternatives. Nai Zindagi in Pakistan, for example (see page 13), has created mixed residential and commercial communities on the outskirts of Islamabad and Lahore, whereby stabilised drug users can move into environmentally friendly houses built by their peers, learn a trade in nearby workshops and continue to access treatment and support as they build a new life centred around the usual pastimes of work, families and leisure. Mukti Sadan, in Mumbai in India (see page 26), runs industrial units which give recovering users structured vocational training and helps them escape the worst aspects of the largest slum in the world (where drug use is rife) into jobs and non-using communities.

To create belonging

The second priority is to help people find a sense of belonging. Some find a sense of community in the shared bond of being stigmatised by the mainstream. But their long-term survival depends on breaking out of the homogeneity of the drug user community and accessing wider social networks.

Mukti Sadan, for example, engages women from across the drug using and non-using communities in printing workshops, and even runs schools for their children in order to build the confidence and understanding among both groups to live and work together. Kaleidoscope (see page 55), serving south west London, delivers the widest lifelong learning provision in the Royal Borough of Kingston through its Tutors' House. It attracts two thirds of its students from the wider community (including school refusers referred by the local education authority) as well as a third from its drug treatment services. It is currently working with award-winning architects and engineers to create a state of the art learning centre which will heighten the project's appeal to all-comers due to the quality of its ICT and business suites, fine art and digital graphics studios and professional music recording studio. Sharan, in Delhi (see page 39), ensures its specialist treatment services are just one part of a broad spectrum of primary health care accessible to the whole community.

To resolve trauma

The third priority is to tackle the traumas and loss. The Forum projects offer the usual range of counselling services, but they also work hard at extending hospitality and warmth which help people secure new attachments, and offer new ways of making sense of their lives. In contrast to the rather clinical waiting rooms and appointment protocols of traditional treatment settings, they excel at creating spaces where clients feel at home. Numerous relationships and marriages have flourished because staff make introductions and help clients form new connections through the day to day life of the project. The sense of brotherhood among staff and clients alike is noticeable. This will strike many practitioners as distinctly odd, but when you consider that the alternative for many is the persecution of the streets (for example, in north east India members of insurgency groups drive padlocks through the ears of users to indicate they are marked men and will be shot if they don't quit using) it makes evident sense.

To provide alternative allies and occupations
The Forum projects act as gateways to new social and employment networks which seemed far beyond the reach of their clients even before their drug use became a problem. When clients at Sahara (see page 46) are ready to move into a range of businesses they run in Delhi and other sites across India, for example, their neighbours get to know them only as the person who prints their annual report in the print shop or makes a letter rack to order as a gift for a friend. This is a powerful experience which underscores the redemptive power of work. It is hard to overstate the long held lack of confidence of many dependent drug users.

Enterprise and self-sufficiency
Many of these methods can be relatively expensive. Given the absence of consistent funding from government it has therefore been essential to find ways for them to pay their own way. Necessity forced the Forum organisations to develop a hard nosed business sense, but also as Tariq Zafar, who founded and runs Nai Zindagi, points out, too often NGOs simply reflect the dependency of their clients in their relationships with funders. Developing successful enterprises with real markets has also been crucial in helping their clients engage with the real world.

To promote optimism and opportunity

Given that the sense of a blocked future is so profoundly shaped by larger economic and social factors, this last factor is the hardest to tackle. But the Forum projects have worked hard to find ways of fostering optimism by providing skills and career opportunities, practical work experience in growing enterprises, strong friendships and commitments. Similar considerations apply in the developed world. An improved CV and any amount of job preparation are not going to help a drug user with over 50 convictions and a 15 year gap in their work record persuade an employer sitting on the other side of the desk in an interview that they are the right person for the job. Yet a track record of work, a portfolio, an employer's reference and the opportunity to prospect for jobs through professional networks can succeed, when coupled with the right skill set and attitude. This approach is already yielding results in Kaleidoscope's web based enterprise, where graduates are moving into full time work and university.

That sense of optimism is also encouraged by the power of example. The high proportion of former and stable drug users among the staff of these projects (in some of the Asian projects this is something like 80 per cent) shows that it is possible to change your life irreversibly, providing a daily challenge to the feelings of hopelessness that many drug users experience.

In summary, what makes the Forum projects distinct from the rest of the treatment sector is their vision and ambition for their clients. Their aim is not to help clients drug problems, but to help clients change their lives.

Why the Asian approach can work in the UK

Many will doubt the relevance of the Asian experience to the UK. To them the differences between our respective settings, customs and institutions seem too great.

But for all the reasons outlined above we can feel confident many of the lessons transfer. Besides, the Asians' approach has it roots in the UK and is still being practised in the work of the Kingston-based Kaleidoscope Project today. Also, as we have seen, there is a range of new institutions taking shape in the UK which could form a powerful alliance for change: the National Treatment Agency, the Neighbourhood Renewal Unit, Job Centre Plus and the Youth Justice Board. The real problem in transferring these lessons has more to do with the specific character of the UK scene:

- a debate which still undervalues hard evidence and is preoccupied with questions of law;

- poor mechanisms for spreading good practice;

- overpowerful professional interests;

- rigid structures of local government and health provision.

The next chapter therefore turns to how these barriers can be overcome and what other steps we should consider now that the drug problem affects nations everywhere.

Case study: Kaleidoscope

The affluent London suburb of Kingston-upon-Thames is the unlikely setting for Kaleidoscope, one of the largest independent drug treatment centres in the UK. The core of the project is a methadone treatment programme. But this is essentially a way of helping people to stabilise their lives so that they can go onto make use of a wide range of other services – from education to job preparation.

Drug users are not the only clients. Kaleidoscope also supports asylum seekers, the elderly, school refusers, the long-term unemployed and people with mental health difficulties. But it is best known for its radical approach to drugs, which starts from a passionate commitment to helping the most marginalised.

Kaleidoscope set up what is now Britain's only open access 'wet' centre for chaotic street users. The project recognises that appointments, mandatory registrations and locked doors can all get in the way of reaching the most excluded. Having engaged users, the project is rigorous about personalising support – encouraging clients to address their underlying problems before trying to survive without the pharmaceutical props which currently get them through the day. For example, this might involve dealing with behavioural difficulties, a literacy problem, debt or an unresolved issue with their family.

The project makes the greatest departure from the normal treatment models with its emphasis on learning and employment. The project's Tutors' House is probably unique in delivering teaching to people who are still spending most of their day chasing a drink or heroin and scraping together enough money to make sure the heating doesn't get cut off at home. It's staff also tutor students in the widest range of subjects anywhere in Kingston – maths and science, music and art, languages and ICT, business, sport and basic skills. The Tutors' House was the first institution to take the government's flagship lifelong learning scheme Learn Direct to highly marginalised groups and, a registered examination centre, it last year achieved the highest AS level score in Persian in the country. Former-drug users happily study alongside clients still using drugs, and two thirds of students have had nothing to do with the treatment scene. Children and young people at risk of problem drug use continue their education here when relationships with mainstream schools and pupil referral units have broken down.

Over the last eighteen months, Kaleidoscope's web production company **simplyworks** has begun helping some of the people facing the biggest barriers to employment. Some have reached their thirties and forties with no experience of work and extensive offending records. Others have spent years in treatment. For them, new skills are not enough to gain work. They need to learn the habits of working life, how to function within organisations and minimise the risk of relapse. Prospective employers need the evidence of a track record of work and a business-to-business reference if they are to overlook a lack of formal education and gaping holes in a client's work history. For their part, clients have no confidence there is a place for them in the world of work and need to effectively do a job to know they can do it. **simplyworks** proves that even clients other employment agencies would see as unemployable can get work given enough support and patience, while matching start-up funding from the Employment Service with income from secured sales within nine months of opening for business.

Kaleidoscope's earlier successes inspired many of the other Forum projects to move in a more holistic direction. **simplyworks** is a sign that this earlier influence is being reciprocated.

What it achieves
Because policy-makers and commissioning managers in health and local authorities have shown little interest in the final destinations of treatment recipients they fund, reliable comparative data is hard to find. However, the available proxies have consistently shown that the Kaleidoscope approach works. Over a quarter of clients receiving help for drugs at Kaleidoscope will be involved in learning at some point in their care, and a third have jobs. Over many years the project has achieved hundreds of successes, helping people to find and keep jobs, homes and partners, and avoid the revolving door syndrome of so much treatment services.

Kaleidoscope is also cost effective and highly practical. As an offshoot of a church, the project pays no rent and benefits from operating out of a public building. Without the usual planning restrictions, the dispensary and needle exchange are open from 7am to 10pm six days a week, where most drug agencies are open during working hours, which makes it hard to combine treatment with a job. Furthermore, these services cost the taxpayer a tenth of the cost charged by local pharmacists. The project mobilises many volunteers, attracting a mix of trained doctors and social workers as well as non-specialists on annual placements.

The Kaleidoscope model has been widely acknowledged. Mike Trace, formerly deputy drugs tsar and now head of performance at the National Treatment Agency has said that "Kaleidoscope delivers the things we dream about in our ivory towers" and many others in the profession have acknowledged its unique contribution.

Kaleidoscope provides a one-stop service – with everything available under one roof. For users it provides a community as much as a service. While many drug agencies limit opportunities for drug users to 'congregate' Kaleidoscope deliberately aims to bring a return to normalcy in drug users' lives through cultivating a supportive social environment in the project's club and its Tutors' House.

That strong sense of community is combined with a very outward looking ethos which enables the project to take ideas from many different sources and work with others – for example, the project is currently collaborating with the housing, social services and mental health teams in the area to ensure lapsing drug users become a statutory housing priority, rather than risking a return to the streets.

And it has a bold creative streak, turning its hand to anything that will engage, motivate and progress its clients – whether that's web design, social enterprise, setting up an independent record label or running an internet café.

7. The way forward for the UK

What lessons should the UK learn from the rapidly evolving international debate? And what should be done to get a grip on problem drug use?

A good starting point is rigour about the goals we are trying to achieve. The former drugs tsar Keith Hellawell often said his goal, shared by many, was a drug free world. For better or worse that is a goal which produces more incredulity than inspiration. No known society in the past has been drug free and it is highly unlikely that any will be in the future. A far more sensible goal is a society in which substance use is well managed, and the risks minimised.

In the past it has been hard to draw constructive distinctions between problem use – of licit as well as illicit drugs and moderated use which is less likely to cause harm. Policy development has been held up. Fortunately this is starting to change. David Blunkett as Home Secretary has markedly shifted the tone of government statements. Other ministers elsewhere in government, not just in domestic departments but also in international ones, should be contributing as well. All need to acknowledge that drug use is pervasive, drug users are not beyond redemption, problem drug use is not insoluble, legal issues are important but not all-important, and that this is a field in which all nations can learn from each other.

This chapter sets out the practical steps that are now needed to form the basis for a more serious, and rounded, approach to drugs:

- a focus on causes, not symptoms;

- an holistic approach to drugs in which work is key;

- social enterprise playing a central role;

- ensuring that the law contributes to the reduction of harm;

- action to tackle the barriers to change;

- a concerted approach at the global level to deal with the causes and effects of drugs;

- effective lesson learning.

1. Focus on causes – not symptoms

Policy focused on symptoms is bound to fail. Greater gains are to be had more cost effectively when policy addresses causes, not symptoms. This is big lesson for social policy more generally and it has been applied well in other fields. For example, homelessness agencies understand well that providing housing is not a sufficient solution for homelessness. Teenagers and their families need support before a breakdown, men leaving prison need help adjusting to life outside, while rough sleepers often need help with drink and drug problems as well as somewhere to sleep at night. Yet so impoverished is the debate about drugs that we have barely grasped the point in this field. A more mature approach to drugs would involve some of the following:

A national anti-drug strategy re-framed around a holistic analysis and measurable outcomes. The current strategy is flawed on two counts. Its targets which focus on reductions in use of cocaine and heroin, general use among young people and rises in seizures – are misconceived. Even if they were the right targets the lack of either baseline data with which to measure progress, or of serious analysis of likely trends, would render them next to useless.

If we were instead to build on what we know about problem use, the strategy would aim to end the revolving door of treatment by supporting long-term change in users' lives and ensuring young people at risk receive help in making the transition to independence before they develop an entrenched drug habit. It would target in particular the number of problem users, rates of relapse, the rate at which young people become newly dependent and the concentrated street availability of drugs.

A more rounded approach would keep the focus on harm reduction. Innovations to cut waste of police and court time – like the Lambeth cannabis trials – would be followed up. Other measures to reduce harm might include the introduction of licensed venues for the safe consumption of drugs, vending machines for needles and syringes (as piloted in Australia) and facilities for testing the purity of supplies at petrol stations and other 24 hour venues, and tasking dance clubs to teach drug-related first aid. Schools could be encouraged not simply to exclude children for using drugs, but to ensure they receive help in taking control of their lives. In all of these examples the key should be to reward innovation and outcomes not professional vested interests.

Stop spending money on drugs education which achieves nothing. One more controversial result of a much more rigorous focus on outcomes and evidence would be an end to much drugs education. This now takes up a large slice of the drugs budget but with little or no evidence that it is effective, and strong anecdotal evidence that pupils treat it with contempt.

Drug policy should no longer be centred around types of drug. Instead it should be shaped by the hierarchy of harms evident in different patterns of drug use. Single issue campaigns – against, for example, solvents falling into the hands of teenagers least able to judge their dangers, or a sudden influx of contaminated heroin – will always play an important role. But long-term the biggest impact will come from measures which deal with patterns of drug use, not specific drugs: in other words dealing with people rather than substances, and linking drug policy much more explicitly to social and employment policy.

2. Adopt an holistic approach in which work is key

Treatment has a role, but all the causes of addiction need to be tackled, not just medical ones, if people's lives are to be changed. Many drug dependents need treatment because without help in dealing with the chemistry of addiction it is hard to change lives. But this is not enough. Too much focus on treatment just leads to a revolving door, and a very expensive one.

An increasingly important part of the emerging agenda will be work. Work can serve a genuinely redemptive role for drug users. However, the lead agencies will need to change if they are to help tens of thousands of drug users make the transition from dependency into work. The following are key to better outcomes:

Creating lasting structures for recovery. The creation of the National Treatment Agency (NTA) could be a good opportunity. The risk is that it will revert to a traditional medical model, a risk that is reinforced by its position under the Department of Health. A much better approach would be to focus on outcomes investing in whatever works in helping people to change their lives. That would mean defining it in terms of the outcomes it should achieve, not in terms of treatment which is effectively an input. It would be renamed as the National Drugs Rehabilitation Agency, and it would spend money and energy on a range of actions of which treatment will be just one. Education, work, enterprise, community building would all be on its menu.

Whether or not this can happen in the short-term, the NTA should take steps now to integrate work and training into treatment – some UK based agencies, like the Govern Addiction Service, are beginning to share the Forum projects' view that work serves a therapeutic role in the early stages of treatment as well as an exit route from later stages. So for example the majority of drug users entering residential rehabs could do so in their locality so that training, volunteering and work, together with re-housing and follow-on care can all be brought together to make a durable impact where it counts. Prisoners serving sentences for non-violent drug related offences could spend the majority of their time working in on-site businesses.

But responsibility for drugs should not be the exclusive responsibility of the NTA. To reach all those in need of help, it is vital that all statutory services likely to be in contact with marginalised young people such as Connexions or the Employment Service, should be able to identify those at risk of entrenched drug misuse through comprehensive assessment tools like ASSET, developed by the Youth Justice Board. GPs and specialist drug agencies should provide medical treatment to under 16s according to need. Youth custody centres should combine treatment with a central emphasis on training, work and putting practical arrangements in place for the future. Pupil Referral Units, schools and sixth form colleges working in disadvantaged areas should develop stronger, outward-looking work-based strands with the explicit aim of helping young people with weak support networks secure the transition to independence.

Strengthen the links between regeneration and action on drugs. The Neighbourhood Renewal Unit should develop specific work on drugs, and local strategies for dealing with drug markets should be developed under Local Strategic Partnerships in areas where there are acute problems. Given the overwhelming correlation between problem drug use and deprivation, and the relationship between drug use, crime, unemployment and poor public spaces, every area regeneration programme needs to be able to tackle the related problems of dealing, crime and ill-health associated with drugs. Some will need to build alliances with their neighbours since drug markets are no respecters of formal boundaries.

Local commissioning bodies should pool resources to reward 'distance travelled', rather than inputs. In the long run the key to a more outcome focused approach will be money: if funds are simply devoted to inputs, like treatment episodes, the agencies on the ground are unlikely to change. Money should reward success in delivering lasting change (the 'distance travelled' by users) with more money going to agencies which can make progress with the hardest to help clients.

Community organisations need to be involved closely in order to promote the shift of opinion and breadth of support for durable change. The work of Mothers Against Drugs (MAD) in Greater Easterhouse, Scotland, is just one example which shows how a community can respond intelligently to drugs: the death of a 12 year-old supplied with heroin by a dealer on his estate prompted thousands of people to take to the streets in protest. Anger was the first response and led to dealers being harried and chased off estates. But as the group learnt more about the causes of the problem, it recognised that most dealers were addicts who needed help if they were to change their behaviour. Three years on, MAD has become an effective grassroots catalyst, bringing treatment, detox and vocational training to users in its neighbourhood.

Police have a key role to play here too. In many areas officers working at a local level have been at the forefront of thinking more radically, and constructively about drugs, working with other agencies and responding to the evidence. Looking to the future the wider agenda set out here stands most chance of succeeding if much more power and resources are devolved to front-line units.

Develop new ways of helping people into work. The new Job Centre Plus (JCP) agency will need to become much more sophisticated in helping clients to become job-ready. A bit of coaching on job search will not yield results for this group even in times of high employment. Instead the JCP needs to develop better early assessment, and packages that bring together treatment, training and work experience and continuing support from personal advisers. One option would be to combine these in a new set of Treatment and Employment Compacts (TECs) tied into Jobseeker Agreements which would be more enabling than the comparable Drug Testing and Treatment Orders (issued by the courts), providing a guaranteed high level of service in exchange for commitments from the user to undergo treatment and develop skills. A system of nomination rights could be operated which would build stronger bridges with local communities by inviting GPs, specialist treatment agencies and faith groups among others to recommend candidates.

The JCP also needs to build up the capacity of the sector to perform and innovate. That may mean encouraging more private employment agencies to work with drug users, encouraging drug agencies to build up their skills in sophisticated labour market initiatives, funding promising innovations, increasing know-how and purchasing power among district managers, and improving the knowledge base. Employment Zones, the New Deal and intermediate labour markets all offer models for doing this with increasing success. The best take a no-holds-barred approach to how money is spent in order to tackle every single barrier to jobs. That may also mean better links with housing departments to ensure that lack of accommodation does not undermine people's prospects of getting away from addiction to drugs.

Reforming the benefits system to remove the disincentives to work. Drug users taking the first steps in full-time learning, training or work placements risk a drop or stop in income. They can lose housing tenancies and support for childcare and travel to training while their prospects of earning income from legitimate sources are still low. Given their low confidence this puts many off – the typical client of treatment services is over 25, with no experience or large gaps in their track record of work or other constructive occupation, and a criminal record. Benefits assessors need sufficient flexibility to be able to judge their clients' prospects, progress and what will take them forward, rather than imposing sanctions which lead to repeated short term failure. Drug users with related physical or mental health problems, like people with other periodic disabilities such as MS, need a different approach which supports them – and just as importantly their employers – in ways that recognise their ability to function well for large periods of time despite repeated short periods of sickness.

3. Give social enterprise a central role

Statutory agencies tend to deal only with single issues. Social enterprises can be much more effective at bringing together all the services that drug users need to overcome their problems. They are more innovative. And they are more likely to motivate drug users fed up with trying to navigate their way through a bewildering array of advice and suspicious of mainstream provision.

As in Asia social enterprise needs to play a central role in the next stage of drugs policy in the UK, with concerted action to build up a dynamic sector able to solve problems, create jobs and revitalise communities that have been damaged by drugs.

A first step would be to launch a business incubator dedicated to stimulating social enterprises which train and employ long term drug users. Concentrating resources and know-how, the incubator would be tasked with accelerating the growth of specialist enterprises, working in partnership with financial institutions. It might aim in ten years to have supported the creation of around 25,000 jobs, numerous other training and development opportunities and sustained growth within the sector of between four to nine per cent. To achieve this goal, it would:

- champion the role of social enterprise in the dependency to work agenda;

- facilitate 'deep immersion' in the culture and practice of social enterprise through training, exchanges, action learning sets and beacon projects;

- award earmarked start-up funding pooled from all the relevant departments – the Departments of Health, Work and Pensions, Education and Skills, Trade and Industry, and the Home Office – and act as a gateway to relevant mainstream programmes;

- headhunt talent from all sectors to aid delivery;

- act as a conduit for developing good practice – gathering examples, submitting them for peer review, disseminating templates and toolkits, establishing new quality marks;

- provide 'pit-stop consultancy' – these new hybrids combine so many different functions that they need access to advisors who can supply quick answers on the full range of issues they face;

- create a forum for practitioners, drug users and policy makers to align their work and engage in continued debate.

The incubator would itself need to act entrepreneurially by brokering deals between the best performers; encouraging successful models to replicate and identifying franchisees – whether Drug Action Team Co-ordinators, GPs, community workers or entrepreneurs from the commercial sector; creating cost savings by enabling the businesses it supports to share for example marketing, accounting and distribution platforms.

A second step would be to link international good practice on enterprise. An international arm of this incubator is needed to serve a similar purpose for governments, NGOs, businesses and community groups working in producer and distributor communities.

A third would be to identify sectors which offer the best prospect of progress – matching local talent to skills gaps in new or under-resourced industries. In some settings, for example Newcastle, poor transport and inertia can mean drug users seeking work and a sustainable exit strategy from their problems live only a few minutes' travel away from employers who can't fill jobs. Social entrepreneurs or private recruitment agencies like Reed Employment (who have already shown an interest in working with drug users) could be sub-contracted to combine recruitment, training, management, social support, transport, policy and payroll services which serve employers' interests yet meet the needs of drug users. In the public sector, NHS hospitals have begun to show how they can meet the demand for health care workers by working more closely with marginalised communities and helping individuals overcome the barriers that prevent them from applying for vacancies. A North London partnership between the Employment Service and the Employment and Skills Council has adopted a similar approach to fill in vacancies in the gas utilities. These sorts of approaches should be spread.

All three steps would benefit from being affiliated and sharing successes.

4. Ensure the law reduces harm

Sorting out the law on drugs is a necessary but far from sufficient condition for reducing the harm caused by drugs. Current legislation on drugs is widely recognised to be failing: it effectively criminalises many millions, but does little if anything to reduce harm caused by drugs. Developments in Europe and in policy among opposition parties in the UK suggest that change may be imminent – the balance of opinion is moving steadily in favour of a more liberal legal framework.

However, too often changing the law is presented as a panacea for all the problems drugs cause, when clearly it is not. More likely legal change will create both opportunities and new problems: opportunities to treat drugs in a more open and honest way; problems of defining the right way to regulate drug use, to protect children, and ensure that greater availability at potentially lower cost does not create new dangers in its wake.

How for example would we organise regulation and distribution, given the only sensible solutions will need to put some restrictions on use? What should be done about taxation and should new sources of revenue be hypothecated to prevention and treatment? Would a hardcore develop more destructive habits, as some evidence from the Swiss heroin trials potentially implies? What would happen to those at the end of the supply chain who currently live by the informal economy off-register, and would they seek income from new sources, such as tobacco smuggling or the sex industry?

Full-scale legalisation presents a complex challenge for foreign and domestic policy-makers since it would have to be co-ordinated internationally. Full legalisation in one country would raise a host of problematic issues – practical ones of drug tourism, diplomatic and legal ones in relation to trade and supply. Policy reformers in Holland, Belgium and Portugal have effectively chosen to turn a blind eye to the problems of drug trafficking, but full legalisation would require a more sustainable answer.

For all these reasons legal change is not the whole answer. But there are changes to the law that would reduce harm, subject to careful evaluation of their effects, and tend to have been overlooked in the debate to date:

Agencies experienced in working with drug users should be allowed to permit supervised drug taking on licensed premises. These venues would need to differentiate between different types of drug user and build on the experience of coffee shops, dance venues which provide testing facilities, and supervised injecting rooms in Holland, Switzerland and Australia (and latterly Germany, Luxembourg, Spain and Austria). For example, injecting rooms may need to be accompanied by a relaxation of the guidelines on prescribing heroin and injectable methadone, and may only be made available to clients who have not succeeded with alternative prescribing. Holland has demonstrated how these can be both welcoming and safe, more café than clinic. This would represent the first step in bringing drug use into designated areas of the public domain, away from children, where it can be better managed and the problems minimised. These initiatives could serve an important public health role by engaging those who reject other treatment programmes, educating less experienced users, reducing the spread of blood borne diseases and reducing the nuisance factor where users currently consume in inappropriate public spaces, discarding needles behind them. Dedicated childcare facilities would, of course need to be provided and could ensure users' children enjoy access to a full range of health, education and leisure activities.

Stiffer penalties and more police attention should be brought to bear on adults who supply children with drugs. One Scottish study suggested as many as 6 in 10 children with access to illicit drugs procured them from older siblings or family members and the intention here would not be to exacerbate children's difficulties by disrupting families. However, such an offence would send a clear signal, whatever an individual's views on drugs, that there should be no tolerance for supply to children.

Stiffer penalties should be imposed on people who use in front of children or involve them in the handling of drugs. Drug using parents currently have little choice but to use in their own homes where they are least likely to be detected. Those who are householders can come under heavy pressure from homeless friends to keep an open house for other users. Too many children witness traumatic scenes, find themselves around conflict or violence or simply at some point find themselves excluded. The combination of licensed venues for drug use and tougher penalties for involving children would set a valuable new norm. The ban on handling would make it more difficult for dealers to use children as less conspicuous runners and reduce the chances of them being recruited into drug markets longer term. And dealing around schools and play areas would be more heavily penalised.

Drug users should be prosecuted for the irresponsible disposal of contaminated works. Dirty needles and other paraphernalia present a real hazard and their casual disposal presents one of the legitimate complaints against some drug users. This law would make the right distinction between punishing the drug user and punishing inappropriate behaviour. It should be supported by the wider distribution of retractable needles and sharps bins designed to hold needles securely.

Measures of this kind would help to prepare the way for the complex task of regulating drug use in an environment in which drugs themselves might no longer be illegal. They would focus attention on the important issues: how drugs are used, and the harms they cause.

5. Tackle the barriers to change

All our experience tells us that progress is unlikely to happen without a very different style of debate – one based on evidence and reason, not subject to the vagaries of prejudice, blame and vested interests. Without celebrating it, we need to acknowledge the pervasive nature of drug use. For generations among whom drug use is normal it is simply not credible to portray drugs as a marginal evil.

Yet to date too many (radical practitioners, politicians and activists, drug users and the people who try to help them) have in the past found themselves susceptible to threats and abrupt about-turns on policy, their careers and livelihoods at risk. War has repeatedly been declared and a tough line on drugs has blurred into a tough line on drug users. While the tone is beginning to change, greater leadership will be needed if today's appetite for reform isn't all too soon to become yesterday's political suicide.

Cabinet ministers need to publicly sponsor efforts to improve the drug policy environment and encourage us to see the issue more as one of science, less as a matter of opinion. Real leadership requires ministers to broker an informed, open exchange between experts including health and crime professionals, practitioners in regeneration and employment, academics and social scientists. They need to stop allowing commentators and media pundits out for cheap lines to dominate the debate, build consensus based on the evidence, and bring in those with lessons to share, wherever they may be. As the experience of the Social Exclusion Unit has shown, this is better done inclusively. It should not be left solely to the Home Office. Other ministers, from DfID, DTI and FCO, have a role to play too, drawing in the implications for, and lessons from, other fields.

The government, academic and professional bodies and trusts and foundations can support a shift in tone by commissioning more holistic research. This should aim to extend our knowledge of the social significance of problem use, and of the most effective interventions which address the causes of dependent use. One of the effects of moral gagging has been that the drug field is short on adequate analysis and would benefit from much more systematic measurement and investigation. As has happened with educational research, giving more control to frontline practitioners to determine priorities will help ensure the most pressing issues are addressed.

Drug users must themselves be included in the community of knowledge creators. In almost every other field (neighbourhood renewal, youth crime, disability and mental health) the value of involving the people directly affected by a problem in developing greater understanding and generating credible new solutions has been recognised and acted upon. At the moment the drugs field suffers from too many structures and procedures which work against agreed goals. For example, some needle exchanges ration supplies; few treatment agencies open beyond working hours; some expect users to be in control of their drug use before they enter treatment. Engaging drug users in the development and evaluation of policy and practice would quickly eliminate counterproductive measures and increase the potential for greater performance, as the experience of the Asian projects demonstrates.

In order to do this we need to adopt a new language for promoting drug users' potential. As the Asian projects and American methadone advocates – lawyers, teachers and so on – visibly demonstrate, drug users who regain control of their use have the potential to more than make good the harm they previously did to their communities in their roles as community leaders and social entrepreneurs.

6. Match new domestic policies with a new global approach

This report demonstrates the extent to which drugs are a truly global phenomenon. As we have seen, no sensible distinction can today be made between so-called 'producer' and 'consumer' countries. The drug trade is the world's largest rogue industry against which few effective levers or sanctions are applied. It enjoys an enormous mark-up from the cost of the raw commodity to the eventual retail price. The trade itself is hugely destructive but so are its connections to the arms trade, human rights abuses, death and violence, and the murky economy of tax havens.

Measures of recent decades focused on cutting supply, have been signally unsuccessful. The current Plan Colombia (the largest ever US aid settlement which promised to stem the supply of cocaine into America) may just be the latest expensive failure and another example of US-backed policy that is far too focused on symptoms rather than underlying causes, full of sound and fury but to little effect.

Looking to the future it is vital that changes in policy domestically are matched by a parallel shift of approach globally. There is a similar need for holistic approaches, dealing with all of the causes and a similar need for practical measures to reduce the harms associated with drugs.

In the short-term the international community is likely to concentrate mainly on new ways of co-ordinating the fight against organised crime. A more aggressive approach to regulating offshore tax havens and anonymous bank accounts is long overdue, as are tougher laws on racketeering. However, in parallel, attention needs to be paid to the problems of making two sets of transitions.

We need to help people out of production. This will involve greater investment in strategies for development, crop diversification, creating alternative sources of income, and help for producers and distributors who are often themselves users. The approach of DfID-backed projects where treatment is combined with crop eradication programmes in places like Dir in the North West Frontier Province of Pakistan, have shown that production can be tackled at source in ways that do not further punish the rural poor. However, success is hard to sustain without constant effort, and enforcement, given the huge mark-up for drugs.

In the long term, a more far-reaching transition will be needed. We are only likely to match domestic successes in reducing harm if the world moves in tandem from an illicit industry to a legal, regulated one. Drugs would become another cash crop, to be traded, and in some cases fairly traded. Needless to say such a move would bring with it many complex risks and currently unforeseen consequences. The international community should prepare for these by thinking through alternative scenarios for legalisation, perhaps with commissions of experts along the lines of the Intergovernmental Panel on Climate Change.

7. Ensure that lessons are learnt

Many nations are now experimenting in parallel. All can learn from each other. To that end we need new web-based exchanges to share experiences across national boundaries, to show what works and what doesn't, and to help projects in very different environments lend each other confidence and knowledge. The evolution of the Forum projects has shown that change locally can happen fastest when learning is mutual. Slowly but surely a global community of experiment and mutual support is taking shape: it needs to be built on, supported by a common evidence base, and to straddle the formal knowledge of international agencies and the everyday tacit knowledge of organisations on the street.

Annex: How traditional drug treatment approaches deal with symptoms but cannot address causes

Approach	Interventions	Outcomes	Limitations
Outreach: Youth and community workers, drug workers	Establishes relationships with those not engaged in treatment. Brief counselling, advice. Encourages referrals.	Two-way information exchange. Removes barriers to services. Promotes earlier treatment interventions.	Soft outcomes. Can be undermined by follow-up services with rigid entry criteria, formal relationships or long waiting lists.
Health promotion: Nurses, drug workers	Identifies risk behaviour. Teaches safer injecting, safe sex. Increases drug knowledge and interactions.	Increased knowledge. Raises awareness of treatment options.	Behaviour unlikely to change unless supported by materials - eg clean syringes, condoms – or, among those with entrenched habits, therapeutic learning cycles. Can lack relevance and credibility if message is perceived as instruction or moral judgement. Evidence shows those most at risk are often least able to take up advice.
Needle exchange: Pharmacists, drug workers	Free provision of unlimited clean, disposable needles and syringes, sterilised water and other paraphernalia, sharps bins for safe disposal.	Prevention of transmission of blood borne diseases. Reductions in infections, venal, circulatory and endocrine problems. Protects wider community from discarded needles.	Effectiveness inhibited by constraints on numbers issued per visit, limited range of syringe capacities, lack of accompanying advice, attitude and visibility of some pharmacists, ambivalent policy and funding environment. Doesn't change pattern of consumption.
Counselling: Multidisciplinary teams, accredited counsellors, consultants	Range from brief interventions designed to alleviate crises or build on current motivation for change, through time limited series of structured one to one sessions and intensive psychodynamic models promoting behavioural management. Group work around common issues also popular.	Increased levels of self-esteem, coming to terms with trauma, loss, bereavement and abuse, learning adaptive strategies, enhanced emotional and physical well-being, improved practical strategies around self-management and promoting change, removing barriers to further achievements.	Few counsellors are results oriented, often working within the narrow ideologies of their training. Provides only indirect support for structural change. Terms of engagement can be rigid, particularly failing active drug users.

Dual diagnosis:	Co-ordinate interventions for people experiencing mental health and substance use problems. Sometimes deliver counselling and other services directly.	Help to ensure clients with a dual diagnosis don't fall through the gaps of agencies dealing with only one or other aspects of their care. Strong advocates for needs based services.	Hidebound by limitations of services clients need to plug into. Lack power to fundamentally address flaws in the system.
Substitute prescribing: Consultants, general practitioners	Supplies prescription of opiates with longer half-life. A maintenance regime aims to provide stability and can be enduring, just as insulin programmes can be. A reduction schedule aims to 'wean' users off opiates by tapering the script and stopping use over a period of six to 18 months, although there is a wide range of variation in treatment episodes.	Prevents physical withdrawals, thereby stabilising drug use, reducing involvement in drug markets, proven reduction in crime, improved emotional health, often other health gains. Eases transition to cessation. Buys time to address broader issues, enables heroin dependents to work, bring up families etc.	Doesn't promote change if wider issues aren't addressed and individuals aren't supported in adapting to change. Some evidence UK clinical governance promotes underdosing of methadone; other medications have limited availability and there is no substitute for crack or cocaine. Many regimes aren't needs led. Many continue some use of illicit drugs or lapse when medication is withdrawn. Waiting lists still the norm – as much as 12months in places.
Detoxification: Residential hospital wards, specialist residential detoxes run by the private and voluntary sectors (often attached to rehabs), GPs and other community based drug teams	Medically supervised withdrawal and cessation of all drugs, including alcohol, over a number of weeks. Group and peer support for adapting to change. In theory, planned throughcare.	Respite from chaotic drug use. Quick transition to being drug free. Enables wider medical assessments to be made and gives users opportunity for clear-headed reflection. Lays the foundation for further progress.	Not a change maker in itself – many use again immediately after discharge with higher risk of overdose. Expensive – around £6,000 per visit. Long waiting lists – high drop-out rates even prior to entry. No accommodation of clients needing a maintenance script or wanting a selective detox.
Residential rehabilitation: Multidisciplinary teams, mainly voluntary sector or private	Structured daily routines within drug-free setting over period of 6-12months. Often in two stages: the first supporting change within the individual, the second encouraging some training,	Maintenance of a drug free lifestyle for duration of stay. Personal development. Taste of alternative lifestyles without recourse to drugs. Models of relapse prevention which can be	Institutional setting doesn't enable drug users to cope in an environment where drugs are readily available; don't effect structural changes in home environment which contributed to drug habit.

	work or voluntary placements. Concept houses ask new entrants to work up strict hierarchies. Many adhere to the 12 Step programme. A similar curriculum can be found in structured day programmes.	practised after leaving.	Training and work often low grade, not linked to a client's local labour markets. Some clients struggle with prescriptive regimes. Expensive – around £7.5-15,000 per stay.
12 Step programmes: Drug workers	Systematic approach to understanding drug use and self-management. Demands regular investment in follow-up practices through peer support groups such as Narcotics Anonymous and AA.	Can bring sense of order and control, friendship and strong sense of solidarity with other abstainers. Can help anticipate relapse and promote early re-entry to treatment.	Doesn't suit everyone, often not enough to resolve a crisis – but complements other interventions. Maintains once a drug user, always at risk of becoming one again. Doesn't address structural factors in dependency, or recognise their role in reducing risk to point at which it can be discounted.

Further reading and resources

Advisory Council on the Misuse of Drugs. 1998. *Drug Misuse and the Environment.* Home Office, London. An excellent summary of the data on drugs and deprivation in the UK from which much of the relevant evidence has been taken for this report.

Effective Interventions Unit. 2001. *Moving On: Education, training and employment for recovering drug users.* Scottish Executive. Edinburgh. Available as a PDF download from www.drugmisuse.isdscotland.org/goodpractice/EIU_movingon.htm

Jacobs, B A. 1999. *Dealing Crack: The social world of street corner selling.* Northeastern University Press, Boston. A good example of what ethnography can bring to our understanding of drugs – the bibliography is extensive.

McIntosh, J and McKeganey, N. May 2000. 'The recovery from drug dependent use: Addicts' strategies for reducing the risk of relapse. *Drugs, Education, Prevention and Policy; vol 7, no 2.*

Wilkinson, F. 2001. *Heroin: The failure of prohibition and what to do now.* Centre for Reform, London. A recent overview of the argument for legalisation; see www.transform.org.uk for further debate on the law.

Wilkinson, R. 2000. *Mind the Gap.* Weidenfeld and Nicholson, London. A succinct summary of the impact of economic and social inequalities on health.

For details of interim reports from the National Treatment Outcomes Research Study, contact the National Addiction Centre: 4 Walk, Denmark Hill, London SE5 0AF; tel 020 7836 5454.

For details of making policy on drugs in Western Australia: www.drugsummit.health.wa.gov.au.

For research findings on drugs and social inclusion: www.jrf.org.uk.

The Centre for Economic and Social Inclusion hosts a burgeoning drugs and employment network. To subscribe, send your email address to: mike.stewart@cesi.org.uk.

Also available from The Foreign Policy Centre

Individual publications should be ordered from
Central Books, 99 Wallis Road, London, E9 5LN
tel: 020 8986 5488, fax: 020 8533 5821
email: mo@centralbooks.com

To order online go to www.fpc.org.uk/reports

(Subscriptions are available from the Centre itself)

THE FOREIGN POLICY CENTRE MISSION STATEMENT

March 3rd 1999; Free, with £1 p+p, or free with any pamphlet.

'Likely to be controversial with Mandarins and influential with Ministers', Financial Times

---

THIRD GENERATION CORPORATE CITIZENSHIP:
Public policy and business in society

Simon Zadek
November 2001, £19.95; plus £1 p+p. ISBN 1-903558-08-5
Kindly supported by Diageo and Friends Ivory & Sime

The role of business in society is one of the most important and contentious public policy issues of our age. Simon Zadek argues that for corporate citizenship to work there needs to be a decisive move beyond individual leadership, philanthropic gesture and PR stunts towards collective action with governments and civil society organisation, what he calls Third Generation Corporate Citizenship. The report sets out an agenda for business in society, taking into account the progress of the corporate citizenship debate so far and shows how through a combination of 'sticks and carrots' governments can play a fuller role in developing new alliances that will make globalisation sustainable.

THE PRO-EUROPEAN READER

Dick Leonard & Mark Leonard (editors)
Published by Palgrave
November 2001, £16.99; plus £1 p+p. ISBN 0–333977211

This collection marshals some of the most persuasive arguments in favour of closer European integration. It presents a unique synthesis of political, social and cultural ideas, with essays by Winston Churchill, Jean Monnet, Roy Jenkins, Mikhail Gorbachev and Tony Blair. Moving beyond politics, the collection also includes writers such as Milan Kundera and David Puttnam on the impact of Europe on our everyday lives: from our cities and identities to football and film.

THE FUTURE OF EUROPEAN RURAL COMMUNITIES

Lord Haskins (Policy Brief 3)
July 2001, £2.95; plus £1 p+p. ISBN 1-903558-04-2

Chris Haskins, Chair of the Better Regulation Task Force and Chairman of Northern Foods, argues in this policy brief that there is a unique opportunity for reform of the Common Agricultural Policy in line with the post-Nice agenda and the mid-term evaluation of the Agenda 2000 budget guidelines that will take place next year. He claims that a series of crises in European farming has convinced policy-makers, farmers and the general public that reform is a priority. At the same time the cost of defending the status quo is also becoming increasingly clear – the CAP is blocking a further round of world trade liberalisation that would benefit other sectors of European business.

This policy brief is the launch pad for a major nine-month project on these issues that will report in June 2002.

THE KIDNAPPING BUSINESS

Rachel Briggs
Kindly supported by Hiscox, Control Risks Group, ASM Ltd., Marsh Ltd. and SCR
March 2001, £14.95; plus £1 p+p

This report addresses the risk of kidnapping for UK citizens travelling and working abroad. As more and more UK companies locate overseas, charities get involved in risky areas and the public's appetite for daring tourist destinations increases year on year, this report highlights the confusion in each of the groups about who is responsible for their safety. This report sets out a detailed plan for UK policy makers in government, companies and charities and clarifies their responsibilities, both to their own personnel and to the rest of the policy community. By exploring a preventative approach, based on lowering the opportunities for kidnapping, The Kidnapping Business offers an invaluable insight into tackling other similar cross-cutting issues that require new forms of engagement between actors in the public, private and voluntary sectors.

THE FUTURE SHAPE OF EUROPE

Mark Leonard (editor)
Kindly supported by Adamson BSMG Worldwide
November 2000 £9.95; plus £1 p+p.

An all-star cast map out an alternative vision for the future governance of Europe, looking at politics and legitimacy, economic governance and reform, Europe's values and role in the world. Solutions to the debate are offered by German Foreign Minister Joschka Fischer, British Prime Minister Tony Blair, Italian Premier Giuliano Amato, French Foreign Minister Hubert Védrine and Swedish Foreign Minister Anna Lindh and show that European governments are grappling with the central questions of European reform and legitimacy in a new way.

Leading thinkers including Anthony Giddens, Jan Zielonka, Alison Cottrell, Ben Hall and Mark Leonard look at what a new case for Europe will mean in practice – in economics, Europe's global role, institutional reform and democratisation.

DEMOCRATISING GLOBAL SPORT

Sunder Katwala, The Foreign Policy Centre
September 2000 £9.95; plus £1 p+p. ISBN 0-903558-00-X

'A timely contribution to the debate on the future of sport', **Sir Paul Condon, Director, International Cricket Council Anti-Corruption Unit**

'Excellent, timely and stimulating', **George Walker, Head of the Sport Department, Council of Europe**

NGO RIGHTS AND RESPONSIBILITIES:
A new deal for global governance

Michael Edwards, Director of Governance, Ford Foundation (writing personally)
In association with NCVO
July 2000 £9.95; plus £1 p+p. ISBN 0-9053558-00-X

'Compelling and succinct', **Peter Hain, former Minister of State, FCO**

'Timely and thought-provoking. Mike Edwards writes from considerable and varied experience and this shows in the balance, objectivity, great good sense and flashes of humour which he brings to bear on this important, and too often polarised debate', **David Bryer, Director, Oxfam**

'A smart and insightful account of the changing role of NGOs... a series of excellent policy recommendations', **David Held, LSE**

HOW TO WIN THE EURO REFERENDUM: Lessons from 1975

Robert M. Worcester, Chairman, MORI International
5th June 2000 £9.95; plus £1 p+p. ISBN 0-9535598-5-8

Twenty-five years ago, the British public voted 'Yes' to Europe. Yet the pro-European coalition had to turn around hostile public opinion to win a decisive victory. Bob Worcester looks at the factors that were decisive in the 1975 referendum, and examines the lessons for the Europe debate today.

'The Worcester analysis about what decides referendums makes sense', **Peter Riddell**, **The Times**

'Will rightly encourage the leader to take the plunge', **Hugo Young**, **The Guardian**

DANISH EURO VOTE: Lessons for Britain

Mark Leonard and Mariell Juhlin, The Foreign Policy Centre
Briefing paper: the text can be read on www.fpc.org.uk

'Argues that Britain's pro-Europeans would lose unless they win the political as well as the economic argument', **Patrick Wintour**, **The Guardian**

'The Danish result cannot be shrugged off by pro-Europeans, as The Foreign Policy Centre argued yesterday', **Don MacIntyre**, **The Independent**

'Draws several lessons from the Danish campaign: the importance of public trust; of bad timing in view of the fall of the euro; and of an unconvincing economic argument', **Peter Riddell**, **The Times**

GOING PUBLIC:
Diplomacy for the Information Society (interim report)

Mark Leonard and Vidhya Alakeson
May 16 2000 £9.95; plus £1 p+p. ISBN 0-9535598-7-4

The project is supported by the BBC World Service,
The British Council, and the Design Council.

*'An important new pamphlet...argues that the old ideas of
British diplomacy must change profoundly'*,
Gavin Esler, The Scotsman

*'Argues that diplomacy can no longer simply be pursued at
government-to-government level'*, **Financial Times**

*'Prime Minister Helen Clark said she will look at how the
report's ideas could be adapted to New Zealand'*,
The Christchurch Press

*'The most comprehensive review of British diplomatic
strategy for twenty years...certain to be highly influential'*,
Straits Times, *Singapore*

AFTER MULTICULTURALISM

Yasmin Alibhai-Brown, The Foreign Policy Centre
May 2000 £9.95; plus £1 p+p. ISBN 0-9535598-8-2

Yasmin Alibhai-Brown argues that we need to fundamentally rethink our approach to national identity, race and public culture. The old debate about multiculturalism cannot meet the challenge of reinventing identity and participation in a devolved Britain, a plural Europe and an increasingly interdependent world. We need to leave behind a debate which has too often engaged blacks, Asians and 'ethnic minorities' rather than whites as well. Yasmin shows how we must create new ways of talking about who we are, and what this will mean in specific policy areas, if the coming battles over political culture and national identity are to have a progressive outcome.

RE-ENGAGING RUSSIA

John Lloyd, Journalist and Member of The Foreign Policy Centre's Advisory Council
In association with BP Amoco
20th March 2000 £9.95; plus £1 p+p. ISBN 0-9535598-6-6

'Re-engaging Russia is excellent on where Russia's relationships with the West went wrong...thought-provoking, highly enjoyable, creative and timely',
Rt Hon Keith Vaz MP, Minister for Europe

'Characteristically thoughtful and well-written, the pamphlet by this outstanding journalist and Russia-watcher recognises the failures both of post-Soviet Russia and of western policy towards the country. John Lloyd argues convincingly that the answer is not for the west to disengage Russia but to engage differently',
Prof. Archie Brown, St Antony's College, Oxford

NEW VISIONS FOR EUROPE:
The Millennium Pledge

Mark Leonard, Vidhya Alakeson and Stephen Edwards, The Foreign Policy Centre
In association with Clifford Chance
24th November 1999 £2.95; plus £1 p+p. ISBN 0-9535598-5-8

A proposed commitment from the governments to the peoples of Europe, outlining the approach and policy reforms which could help to reconnect the EU to its citizens.

The full text can be read on www.fpc.org.uk

REINVENTING THE COMMONWEALTH

Kate Ford and Sunder Katwala, The Foreign Policy Centre
In association with the Royal Commonwealth Society
November 1999 £9.95; plus £1 p+p. ISBN 0-9535598-4-5

Launched at the Durban Heads of Government Meeting, this report shows how wide-reaching Commonwealth reform could create a modern, effective and relevant organisation – helping members to thrive in the 21st century by creating an internationally-recognised standard for good governance and the conditions for investment.

'Intelligent and wide-reaching', **The Times**

'[The Centre's report has] very strong merits. Its proposals deserve honest enquiry', **Business Day,** *South Africa*

'My first thought was "Why has it taken 50 years to start this debate? Why aren't more developing countries leading it?"', **Sharon Chetty,** *The Sowetan*

TRADING IDENTITIES:
Why Countries and Companies Are Becoming More Alike

Wally Olins, co-founder of Wolff Olins, branding and identity consultant
October 1999 £9.95; plus £1 p+p. ISBN 0-9535598-3-1

Countries and companies are changing fast – and they are becoming more like each other. As countries develop their "national brands" to compete for investment, trade and tourism, mega-merged global companies are using nation-building techniques to achieve internal cohesion across cultures and are becoming ever more involved in providing public services like education and health. Wally Olins asks what these cross-cutting trends mean for the new balance of global power.

'A fascinating pamphlet', **Peter Preston, The Guardian**

GLOBALIZATION – KEY CONCEPTS, Number One

David Held & Anthony McGrew, David Goldblatt & Jonathan Perraton
April 12th 1999 £4.95; plus £1 p+p. ISBN 0-9535598-0-7

Globalization is the buzz-word of the age – but how many people understand it? In this much-needed concise and authoritative guide, globalization's leading theorists thrash out what it really means, and argue that we need to rethink politics to keep up with the changing shape of power. Globalization launches the Key Concepts series – holding all of the hidden assumptions behind foreign policy up to the light, and unpacking the key terms to find out what they really mean for policy-makers today.

'An indispensable counterweight to optimists and pessimists alike', **Will Hutton**

'This is the agenda on which a new politics must be constructed and new alliances forged', **Clare Short, Secretary of State for International Development, New Statesman**

NETWORK EUROPE

Mark Leonard, The Foreign Policy Centre
In association with Clifford Chance
10th September 1999 £9.95; plus £1 p+p. ISBN 0-9535598-2-3

'A radical agenda for reform from the government's favourite foreign policy think-tank', Stephen Castle, **Independent on Sunday**

'A welcome contribution to the important debate about Europe's future', Rt Hon Tony Blair MP, **Prime Minister**

THE POSTMODERN STATE AND THE NEW WORLD ORDER

Robert Cooper, Cabinet Office (writing in a personal capacity)
In association with Demos
2nd edition

What did 1989 really mean? Robert Cooper argues that the end of the Cold War also marked the end of the balance-of-power system in Europe. Yet today's open, multi-lateral postmodern states must deal with a complex world – where many states follow traditional realpolitik, while collapsed and failing states present the dangers of pre-modern chaos. The second edition of this groundbreaking pamphlet also addresses how the role of religion in international politics is very different today.

'Mr Cooper's pamphlet explains, lucidly and elegantly, how the emergence of what he calls the postmodern state has changed international relations', **New Statesman**

WINNING THE EURO REFERENDUM

edited by Mark Leonard and Tom Arbuthnott
Kindly sponsored by KPMG and Adamson BSMG Worldwide

'Winning the euro referendum' is the most detailed analysis yet of public opinion and the euro. A host of experts probe the true state of public opinion, draw lessons from other referendums across the EU and work out what arguments work with different sectors of society.

The pamphlet is an attempt to shift the debate on Europe and the euro out of the realm of fear and to couch it in terms which people can understand. It sets out the case for winning a euro referendum and in doing so, challenges some of the received wisdom that defines newspaper coverage of opinion polls.

'The most comprehensive study of polling evidence on the issue to date', **Paul Waugh**, **The Independent**

'The most detailed blueprint to date on ways and means of winning the euro referendum', **Matthew d'Ancona**, **The Sunday Telegraph**

Forthcoming Publications

Mark Leonard and Catherine Stead on
Public Diplomacy: Comparative Experiences

Mark Leonard, Sacha Chan Kam and Phoebe Griffith on
Immigration, Integration and Citizenship
(kindly supported by The Employability Forum)

Rachel Briggs on **Travel Advice**

Yasmin Alibhai-Brown, David Blunkett, Michael Wills, David
Lammy, Philip Dodd, Francesca Klug and others on
**Global Britons: Reflections on identity after Oldham,
Bradford and September 11th**

Adrienne Katz on Identity and Young People

Francesca Klug on Human Rights

Need to Know, a novel by Narration

Christopher Haskins on **The Future of European Agriculture**

- See www.fpc.org.uk for news and information.

- Write to mail@fpc.org.uk to join our email list

Subscribe to The Foreign Policy Centre

The Foreign Policy Centre offers a number of ways for people to get involved. Our subscription scheme keeps you up-to-date with our work, with at least six free publications each year and our quarterly newsletter, Global Thinking. Subscribers also receive major discounts on events and further publications.

Type of Subscription	Price
☐ Individuals	£50
☐ Organisations	£150
☐ Corporate and Libraries (will receive ALL publications)	£200

Please make cheques payable to **The Foreign Policy Centre**, indicating clearly your postal and email address and the appropriate package, and send to Subscriptions, The Foreign Policy Centre, Mezzanine Floor, Elizabeth House, 39 York Road, London SE1 7NQ. For further details, contact Rachel Briggs: rachel@fpc.org.uk

The Foreign Policy Centre Diplomatic Forum

The Foreign Policy Centre Diplomatic Forum is aimed at the key embassy players. It is an ideal way for embassies to keep up-to-date with the work of The Foreign Policy Centre and will provide a useful environment for ideas sharing.

Members will receive the following benefits:

- Special invitations to attend The Foreign Policy Centre annual Diplomatic Forum, which will be led by a high-profile speaker, bringing together key embassy players to address one or more of the foreign policy issues of the day

- Three free copies of every Foreign Policy Centre publication

- Three free copies of *Global Thinking*, The Foreign Policy Centre's newsletter

- VIP invitations for up to three embassy representatives to all Foreign Policy Centre public events

- Event reports from major Foreign Policy Centre events and seminars

Membership of The Foreign Policy Centre Diplomatic Forum is £500 per year. For further details, please contact Rachel Briggs, rachel@fpc.org.uk

The Foreign Policy Centre Business Partnership

The Foreign Policy Centre also runs a Business Partnership scheme, which aims to bring the business community to the heart of foreign policy thinking.

For more details about this scheme, please contact Rachel Briggs, rachel@fpc.org.uk

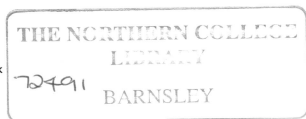